Jordi Nadal was born in Barcelona in 1962 and holds a degree in German Literature from the Universitat de Barcelona. In 2007 he founded Plataforma Editorial.

www.jordinadal.com
www.libroterapia.eu

Book Therapy

Book Therapy

Reading is life

Jordi Nadal

MENSCH PUBLISHING

Original title: *Libroterapia^{TM}*, originally published
in Spanish, in 2017, by Plataforma Editorial.

English-language edition first published in Great Britain 2021 by Mensch
Publishing, 51 Northchurch Road, London N1 4EE, United Kingdom

www.menschpublishing.com

ISBN: PB: 978-1-912914-31-9
eBook: 978-1-912914-32-6

For Clara, who, in February 2017,
said for the first time,
"I can read."

To Xavier Melgarejo, *in memoriam*

"We were put on this Earth to make things."
W. H. Auden (1907-1973)

Contents

Foreword

All humans die, but some books live forever. Every time a book is read, it is transformed into a new creature, understood in a new way, inspiring unexpected reactions. Jordi Nadal's book is by a very rare kind of reader: a publisher. He belongs to that tiny and mysterious group of people who decide which author's scribblings see the light of day. I had the good fortune of having three of my books translated into Spanish by his firm, Plataforma Editorial. It was an extraordinarily wonderful experience.

It showed me how one person's profoundest feelings about what is worthwhile in life can be expressed in a business that knows how to triumph over the merciless realities of earning one's daily bread. I have admired and been moved by his enthusiasm for noble causes, his numerous acts of generosity, his capacity for friendship, his dedication to truth and honesty, and his seemingly inexhaustible energy.

This book gives only a hint of his eclectic, multilingual, international knowledge and tastes. It is unusual in that it reveals how each book he has read has changed and illuminated his own life and ignited a passionate excitement. I am surprised by what he has chosen to emphasise in many of the items on his list of favourite readings. I interpret this as illustrating the impossibility of predicting what effect an author will have on readers, who very often find ideas in a book which are quite different from what the author intended. It is not only authors who give birth to ideas. Every new book one reads, or at least those books that have ideas inside them, may lead to the unexpected birth of an unexpected new thought, a new interest, a new vision of what life is about.

So, book therapy must be distinguished from all other kinds of therapy. It does not diagnose, and it cannot promise a cure. Out of the two million books published each year in the world, many have no other ambition than to put the reader to sleep, or to amuse, or to instruct, or to help pass the time which would otherwise be devoted to fighting against boredom. For me, book therapy means the experience of meeting a stranger. A book is an opportunity to have a conversation with a stranger, a silent conversation which may sometimes continue for years. And though some authors who write many books may sometimes be repeating themselves, others may be evolving, expanding their horizons and discovering new hopes, so that each new book may have been written by a slightly different person. *Book Therapy* is an adventure into the unknown.

THEODORE ZELDIN,
Oxford, March 2021.

Presentation

Why don't you write down the things that you enjoyed reading and which help train managers and leaders; those that also help them become better people?

There began a vital conversation (at least, in the history of this book) with one of the most highly trained managers I know, whose work takes place in one of the most relevant companies in the economic landscape of our country.

I thought for a moment, surprised, disconcerted, flattered… and I accepted the challenge.

And here I tell you why.

In 1978 I began to keep a file on each book I read. I have just under eighteen hundred book reports. I don't count them to show off. It is a fact that is related to my reality, my hobbies, my studies and my profession. Yet despite this, I still never thought that I would start this book.

Since then, I have read, underlined and copied passages that I have enjoyed. Many I remember; some, I reread. My reading is part of my life today – as it is for so many other people – but for me it really is to do with my vocation, my profession and my mission as a publisher.

Books teach us to understand things in a much more profound way than other easy forms of information. In today's world it is not about having more information. More than ever, it is about having criteria, knowing how to select what is relevant. Today it is about knowing how to discard superfluous information and acquire good knowledge.

The poet T. S. Eliot (1888-1965) worded it masterfully in these verses:

"Where is the wisdom we have lost in knowledge?
Where is the knowledge we have lost in information?"

This work is a modest personal guide, a tour of thirty-three authors, to share fragments of those books which were key to me. Therefore, if you would like to enjoy a sample of lucidity and awareness, go ahead. Because I have thought about this as a book to enjoy, as if you had a sweet tooth and went to visit all the best *patisseries* in the world, and from each shop you chose something sweet to allow you to savour the sublime taste of each place. Enjoyment as a superior search method, to learn to manage a little better, with humility and gratitude, your own free life.

It is not about recommending you read books related to creativity or leadership (far from it). Rather, it is about suggesting that you read good literature as a way to access great authors full of knowledge.

Why read good literature?

At least for two reasons.

Let's think back to the film *The Impossible* (Juan Antonio Bayona, 2012). Those seconds, those minutes that follow the terrible tsunami. That terrifying situation where everything is destroyed.

The first thing that is necessary after a flood, whatever its magnitude, is always one simple thing: clean water. Well, our world has been overwhelmed by an internet tsunami, by information overload. To preserve balance, health, harmony and peace, drinking water, pure water, is now necessary, more than ever. Just enough, and nothing more, and above all, filtered.

Reading good things and doing it well is like drinking fresh water in a world full of dirty water, overwhelmed by a flood in which there is an overabundance (as is typical of a flood) of what is mostly very bad, for being trivial, false, or misleading.

Reading good literature is to enjoy something healthy, something wise, something profound, something beautiful, something true. In short, reading well is taking care of your health, as can be seen in the article, "People who read books live up to two years more, according to a study" (*El Mundo*, 5/08/2016).

"The study carried out by three scientists from the School of Public Health of the prestigious American university [Yale] has found that, from the group of readers who have been monitored over 12years, those who spent about three and a half hours reading per week were 17% less likely to die, while those who exceeded these hours of reading reached 23%.

One of the authors of the study, Becca R. Levy, revealed to The New York Times: "People who read a book for as little as half an hour a day have a significant survival advantage," and furthermore, she added that these improvements are not limited to longevity. There are also benefits "for their health, education, cognitive abilities and many other variables."*

According to this study, we read not only to give more longevity to our lives. We also read to give it more depth, more meaning and more intensity.

If the first reason I presented has the drama and force of a tsunami, there is a second reason which is more beautiful, refined, delicate and profound:

> *"Between two doctors whose medical qualifications are otherwise equal, we should trust the one who reads Chekhov."*
> SIMON LEYS (1935-2014)

Let's say we have to be operated on by a surgeon. If both surgeons are just as good as the other, yet there is one who gets excited reading Anton Chekhov (1860-1904), we will be

---

* <www.elmundo.es/f5/2016/08/05/57a3756a46163fc63e8b462b.html>.

less alone with the latter on the operating table. Anyone who has read and been moved by Chekhov (or with another like-minded author, despite there being so few at his level) will have a depth of perspective that will make them a better person, and therefore a better surgeon. Or a better baker, better parent, better musician, better child… Almost certainly: whatever it is, a better one. Because they will have touched on the essence of the question, they will have felt the nuance of it; they will have faltered, and they will have brought out the best version of themselves, because beauty and truth, among other things, are necessary. Because they transform us.

Another reason behind leisurely reading is that it is incompatible with speed, as suggested in the article "Books are not in a hurry" (*El País*, 07/28/2016). Fernando Valverde, secretary of the Spanish Booksellers Guild and the bookseller interviewed for this article, reminded us: "The demand for hurriedness doesn't work with books; books require a slow pace, a return to pleasure. Hurriedness and reading do not go together."[*]

Relaxed reading (literary reading, not the more practical, more opportunistic, utilitarian literature) brings intensity and depth, thereby creating the conditions to achieve a certain serenity. It is something that comes to be of great use in our lives – ever more so as it happens. We live in an age that encourages a form of speed reading that, like channel hopping, is harmful to the soul because it is like sliding over thin ice.

As Ralph W. Emerson (1803-1882) said:

---

[*] <cultura.elpais.com/cultura/2016/07/27/actualidad/1469642158_398059.html>.

"In skating over thin ice, our safety is in our speed."

It is time to stop and think, to feel, to be aware. To be in the here and the now. Less is more, and this also applies to reading and information. We read – when we read well – things that are of a higher quality and which are better. The best reading material makes us better. Or less bad.

It is useful to remember the reflection made by my bookseller friend, when a young man, in his early twenties, a humble and prudent reader, explained to her that he was afraid to go into some bookshops since he was ashamed that someone would notice that he did not read much. The response of the bookseller was as simple as it was enlightening, "There is no possible initiation without education, and a bookshop may well be a school towards knowledge through its books and its authors."

Read as an act of freedom. By making a choice, we actively shape a way to manage our own lives. Reading good books teaches us to live with the contradictions of existence, it teaches us the ways to deal with them without suffering from schizophrenia.

It should be added: books do not allow opportunism. The true life, the one that is our own, which is not borrowed from anyone, does not allow opportunists. The crises that living entails are not resolved by going out to buy something good to read at the last minute. The extinguisher with those essential ideas and feelings which we need to defend ourselves, must gradually fill up with the solemn, silent, intimate and humble nakedness of time and thought.

Some of those reads, in my case after almost forty years of searching, are collected here, in a small book, the result of a life which has been immersed, worked and articulated every day as a reader, editor and, finally, as a person – which is what counts the most. A book that is, furthermore, published coinciding with the tenth anniversary of Plataforma Editorial, a project that was born with the same spirit of promoting good literature with texts that exude **authenticity** and **meaning**, the mantra of the work that I have been publishing in Plataforma Editorial for ten years.

These pages are a way of sharing a reading life that, if it were described through a very illustrative kind of poem, it would say:

To read is to understand.
To understand is to accept.
To accept is to love.
To love is to be.
To be is to achieve.

To achieve is to put living in search of
balance and meaning into practice.

Words make you more of a person,
we learn from differences.
Empathy is the daughter of curiosity.

We learn from differences.
To read is to be more than you could ever wish for.
To understand is to love.
To lead your life is to look for the effective and the affective.

To love is to find meaning.
To read is to move forward.

And with this beautiful idea by Juanjo Millás, I begin the book, and invite you to join me.

> *"Reality is made of words,*
> *so that whoever dominates words,*
> *dominates reality."*
> JUANJO MILLÁS (B. 1946)

Who this work is aimed at:

- People who want to (re)discover the enormous power of literature in ordering, completing and framing their lives. People who want to live with authenticity and meaning.

- Professionals who work with people (in charge of them or as clients) and who want to learn more about the enormous inspirational, stimulating, liberating and meaning-creating power of some of the best literary works.

- People who want to know more about literature, but who perhaps are a little worried about everything they do not know. People who show interest in it and who wish to cultivate themselves, but who are uncomfortable not knowing enough about classics or good modern books.

- People who want to live longer. In this sense, we recommend reading the article "At last a good drug for health: reading lengthens life" (*El País*, 08/22/2016).[*]

In short, this book responds to a legitimate need to satisfy people who seek to savour the experiences and thoughts of some great authors of literature.

---

[*] <elpais.com/elpais/2016/08/19/opinion/1471621596_718582.html>.

Know how to live before dying
Mitch Albom

a. WHO IS MITCH ALBOM?

Mitchell David "Mitch" Albom, born in Passaic, New Jersey, in 1958, is a writer, journalist, screenwriter, playwright, radio host, television presenter and musician. After a career dedicated principally to sports journalism, he established himself as the author of several books, of which have sold more than twenty-six million copies around the globe.

He is known worldwide for his book *Tuesdays with Morrie*, in which he narrates his experiences with Morrie Schwartz, his former mentor, who is suffering from amyotrophic lateral sclerosis (ALS).

Context: United States in the 1990s. In 1995, a great journalist saw his former teacher, Morrie Schwartz, who was suffering from ALS, on a television programme talking about life and death. From that moment on, Albom re-established contact with his old tutor, visiting him at his home every Tuesday to discuss these two important issues.

Our author, looking for a way to bear Schwartz's medical costs, found a publisher willing to publish the book in which he recounts these periodic meetings with his professor, and dedicated his advance to paying for the expensive treatment.

Tuesdays with Morrie was published in 1997 and spent four years on *The New York Times* best-seller list. In addition, more than fourteen million copies have been sold and it has been translated into forty-one languages. In 1999 the book was adapted for television by Mick Jackson, with the wonderful Jack Lemmon as Morrie.

b. FRAGMENTS OF HIS WORK

"'Well, my friend,' he said, 'what are we talking about today?'
'How about family?'

'Family.' He mulled it over for a moment. 'Well, you see mine, all around me.'

He nodded to photos on his bookshelves, of Morrie as a child with his grandmother; Morrie as a young man with his brother, David; Morrie with his wife, Charlotte; Morrie with his two sons, Rob, a journalist in Tokyo, and Jon, a computer expert in Boston.

'I think, in light of what we've been talking about all these weeks, family becomes even more important,' he said.

'The fact is, there is no foundation, no secure ground, upon which people may stand today if it isn't the family. It's become quite clear to me as I've been sick. If you don't have the support and love and caring and concern that you get from a family, you don't have much at all. Love is so supremely important. As our great poet Auden said, 'Love each other or perish.'"

c. BRIEF COMMENTARY

Tuesdays with Morrie is a *vade mecum* of life's big issues. The family occupies a central place in all intimate and sincere conversation, at least for those who have chosen it to be that way.

When a person nears his or her end, they are usually only interested in the essentials. They manage their time and their knowledge, the way they feel and how they breathe, and they put it at the centre of what is important. In everyday language it is usually summed up with a colloquialism like: "Enough of the nonsense."

Tuesdays with Morrie is a wonderful handrail on the staircase of life. It will always be there to give you support.

d. EVERYDAY REFLECTIONS

Write the following words in order of priority: *Work* and *family*. *Family* and *work*. One in first position; the other, in second. You don't have to show anyone. Answer honestly. Your answer is your identity, it is who you are. Moreover, it is who you want to be.

In life we have principles and interests.

Reading this book will allow you to enlighten yourself and to adapt your life's priorities to reality.

e. OTHER RELEVANT FRAGMENTS

"This book was largely Morrie's idea. He called it our 'final thesis.' Like the best of work projects, it brought us closer together, and Morrie was delighted when several publishers expressed interest, even though he died before meeting any

of them. The advance money helped pay Morrie's enormous medical bills, and for that we were both grateful.

*The title, by the way, we came up with one day in Morrie's office. He liked naming things. He had several ideas. But when I said, 'How about **Tuesdays with Morrie**?' he smiled in an almost blushing way, and I knew that was it.*

After Morrie died, I went through boxes of old college material. And I discovered a final paper I had written for one of his classes. It was twenty years old now. On the front page were my pencilled comments scribbled to Morrie, and beneath them were his comments scribbled back.

Mine began, 'Dear Coach…'

His began, 'Dear Player…'

For some reason, each time I read that, I miss him more.

Have you ever really had a teacher? One who saw you as a raw but precious thing, a jewel that, with wisdom, could be polished to a proud shine? If you are lucky enough to find your way to such teachers, you will always find your way back. Sometimes it is only in your head.

Sometimes it is right alongside their beds.

The last class of my old professor's life took place once a week, in his home, by a window in his study where he could watch a small hibiscus plant shed its pink flowers. The class met on Tuesdays. No books were required. The subject was the meaning of life. It was taught from experience.

The teaching goes on."

f. SUGGESTED READING

Tuesdays with Morrie, New York, Doubleday, 1997.

A stoic emperor as an
admirable life model
Marcus Aurelius

a. WHO IS MARCUS AURELIUS?

The Roman emperor and philosopher, Marcus Aurelius Antoninus Augustus (Rome, AD 121-180) was one of the most admired Roman emperors in history. Fatherless from the age of three, when he came to the throne, Marcus Aurelius always claimed that his mother had taught him that it was possible to live without ostentation: "Simplicity in my way of living, far removed from the habits of the rich". It was the Emperor Hadrian who discovered the potential of Marcus Aurelius. Before assuming the throne as emperor, he received the title of Caesar, and was also a consul. Called "the Sage" for his great cultural and philosophical training, marked by stoicism, his uniqueness lies in the fact that throughout his life he devoted himself to writing reflections and thoughts whilst endlessly fighting against the Parthians and the barbarian people.

He became emperor in 161, a position he held jointly with Lucius Verus, Antoninus' other adopted son. From 169 to 177 he ruled alone, and from that year until 180 he did so with his son Commodus, due to the health problems that afflicted him. At the end of his time, in the intervals between the wars against the barbarians of Germania and the Danube border, he devoted himself to writing his ***Meditations*** in Hellenistic Greek. Marcus Aurelius became ill from the plague that ravaged his empire. His son Commodus had to assume command. The emperor died in 180 of smallpox.

Context: Marcus Aurelius is considered one of the most representative figures of Stoic philosophy. Under the protection of Emperor Hadrian, who affectionately called him *verissimus* ('honest'), we are faced with a rare example of enormous power and solid reflective depth, something of great topical relevance, for its unusuality and vitalness, today and forever.

Marcus Aurelius had an empire which faced huge threats: on one hand, in part of Asia, and on the other, in northern Europe, with the barbarians and the Danube border. Although the two fronts always demanded the emperor's full attention, there was a moment in history when the emperor knew and wanted to continually think and reflect on the meaning of power and of life. Although today we are not exactly dealing with the Parthians or the barbarians as imperial enemies, other challenges and dangers surround us. Therefore, his reflections accompany us, guide us and defend us from all the threats that we face.

b. FRAGMENTS FROM HIS WORK

"From my grandfather Verus I learned good morals and the government of my temper.

From the reputation and remembrance of my father,

modesty and a manly character.

From my mother, piety and beneficence, and abstinence, not only from evil deeds, but even from evil thoughts; and further, simplicity in my way of living, far removed from the habits of the rich.

From my great-grandfather, not to have frequented public schools, and to have had good teachers at home, and to know that on such things a man should spend liberally.

Friends, without being either humbled by them or letting them pass unnoticed.

From Sextus, a benevolent disposition, and the example of a family governed in a fatherly manner, and the idea of living conformably to nature; and gravity without affectation, and to look carefully after the interests of friends, and to tolerate ignorant persons, and those who form opinions without consideration: he had the power of readily accommodating himself to all, so that intercourse with him was more agreeable than any flattery; and at the same time he was most highly venerated by those who associated with him: and he had the faculty both of discovering and ordering, in an intelligent and methodical way, the principles necessary for life; and he never showed anger or any other passion, but was entirely free from passion, and also most affectionate; and he could express approbation without noisy display, and he possessed much knowledge without ostentation."

"Begin the morning by saying to thyself, I shall meet with the busy-body, the ungrateful, arrogant, deceitful, envious, unsocial. All these things happen to them by reason of their ignorance of what is good and evil. But I who have seen the

nature of the good that it is beautiful, and of the bad that it is ugly, and the nature of him who does wrong, that it is akin to me, not only of the same blood or seed, but that it participates in the same intelligence and the same portion of the divinity, I can neither be injured by any of them, for no one can fix on me what is ugly, nor can I be angry with my kinsman, nor hate him, for we are made for co-operation, like feet, like hands, like eyelids, like the rows of the upper and lower teeth. To act against one another then is contrary to nature; and it is acting against one another to be vexed and to turn away."

c. BRIEF COMMENTARY

This discourse on applied serenity is divided into twelve books. In the first, which is impressive and admirable in every way, he tells the story of family and friends (and mentions what virtues he has learned from each of them), while the last is a farewell to life. We should take note of this generosity, which speaks much of his greatness.

Nietzsche, who was not easily impressed, recognised the Emperor Marcus Aurelius as a "tonic" for life.

His ***Meditations*** are part of one of the most impressive documents of sincerity in the constant and attentive search for harmony between oneself and human nature. Let's say that when a great power expresses himself in such a deep, human and delicate way, we are in the presence of a beautiful moment in the human condition. There are reasons for hope.

d. EVERYDAY REFLECTIONS

In this world of the powerful, apprentices of belittled and belittling tyrants, deplorable characters who, through tweets and executive orders, generate hatred and yet more hatred, not to mention the chat show hosts and the millions of trolls, there is a need for examples of great people who are not destroyed by the *Hybris*, as the Greeks described it: the arrogance of the mighty.

Emperor Marcus Aurelius gives us cause for hope. If an emperor like him existed, why should we not believe that our lives can be marked by the happy fortune of meeting others like him, be they emperors or, more modestly, key politicians or presidents for example; or, within the world of business, CEOs or Managing Directors? People who help others to live better.

e. OTHER RELEVANT FRAGMENTS

"What is badness? It is that which thou hast often seen. And on the occasion of everything which happens keep this in mind, that it is that which thou hast often seen. Everywhere up and down thou wilt find the same things, with which the old histories are filled, those of the middle ages and those of our own day; with which cities and houses are filled now. There is nothing new: all things are both familiar and short-lived."

"Be not ashamed to be helped; for it is thy business to do thy duty like a soldier in the assault on a town. How then, if being lame thou canst not mount up on the battlements alone, but with the help of another it is possible?"

"What then is that which is able to conduct a man? One thing and only one, philosophy."

"Be thou erect, or be made erect."

"He will live without either pursuing or flying from death."

"The art of life is more like the wrestler's art than the dancer's, in respect of this, that it should stand ready and firm to meet onsets which are sudden and unexpected."

"It is a ridiculous thing for a man not to fly from his own badness, which is indeed possible, but to fly from other men's badness, which is impossible."

"Men exist for the sake of one another. Teach them then or bear with them."

"Do not act as if thou wert going to live ten thousand years. Death hangs over thee. While thou livest, while it is in thy power, be good."

"That which is not good for the swarm, neither is it good for the bee."

f. SUGGESTED READING

Meditations, London, Penguin Classics, 2006.

The value of compromise
Albert Camus

a. WHO IS ALBERT CAMUS?

Albert Camus, a French novelist, playwright, journalist and thinker, was born in Mondovi, in French Algeria, in 1913, into a family of immigrants with limited economic resources. He died at an early age, in Villeblevin, France, in 1960, the victim of a car accident, three years after receiving the Nobel Prize for Literature. His life was an example of lucidity, humanity, tenderness and heartbreak. His biography highlights the power exercised over him by a teacher who believed in his talent, facilitated his access to studies and opened the door to the great world of artistic creation.

Context: Camus is a *pied-noir*. He lived forlorn, but through his journalism he was always fighting the injustices of the Second World War. In Paris, the *apparatchiks* of power, led by Jean-Paul Sartre (1905-1980), tried to crush him. They are barely spoken of, with some exceptions, such as Sartre himself, but Camus survives, stronger than ever.

b. FRAGMENTS OF HIS WORK

"The only way to fight the plague is with decency."

c. BRIEF COMMENTARY

To read Camus is to encounter the light of a transparent and lucid man, human and earthly, whose commitment is to human beings and not to abstract ideas. He has a famous phrase, in which he points out that if he is given the choice between justice and his mother, he would choose his mother, since he could never have forgiven a terrorist – who fights for supposedly greater freedoms and just causes than those of others – blow up a market where other mothers are shopping.

Sartre's resources and all his party influence wore down this rebellious man, a thousand times superior in dignity and goodness to the bureaucrat of communism and the French intelligentsia installed in power and the high life.

His untimely death left us with an unfinished novel, **The First Man**, which is one of the greatest works ever written, examining the fact that human perfection is incomplete.

I discovered Camus reading **The Plague**. It is an essential work on human dignity and on our ability to fight for something that is just. The life of this lonely and loyal man shines light on any moment of doubt. Nobody knew how to suffer like he did. Your life cannot be the same after reading it.

d. EVERYDAY REFLECTIONS

Faced with the absurdity of any unfair situation, the answer is always to fight. A patient and determined fight that comes from waiting, from having hope. Showing solidarity towards other beings and never ignoring the value of human tenderness. Fight at all times, even if death is on the horizon. Always do it, so as not to be accustomed to despair. Nothing should become fossilised, as León Felipe (1884-1968) would also tell us.

Seek. Pursue. Be persistent. Desire and don't allow injustice to make advances. Don't be a parasite or become plagued. Don't allow yourself to be naive or cynical. Camus is the commitment to honesty. Loving (or fighting for the right) must always be a decision.

e. OTHER RELEVANT FRAGMENTS

"Our task as humans is to find the few principles that will calm the infinite anguish of free souls."

"The main thing is not to despair."

"Here I understand what is meant by glory: the right to love without limits."

"'Your victories [doctor] will never be lasting…'
'Yes, I know that. But it's no reason for giving up the struggle.'"

"There are more things to admire in men than to despise."

"The habit of despair is worse than despair itself."

"It is about men of action also being men of ideals; and poets, industrialists. It is about living without dreams, of taking them to action. Before, you either gave up on them or they became lost. They must not be lost or given up on."

"The temptation shared by all forms of intelligence: cynicism."

"Neither fear nor hatred, this is our victory!"

"My life has no worth. What counts are the reasons for my life. I am not a dog."

f. SUGGESTED READING

The First Man, New York, Vintage International, 1996.
The Plague, New York, Penguin Random House, 2002.
Obras completas, ('Complete Works') unavailable in English.
Breviario de la dignidad humana ('Breviary of Human Dignity'), edited by Elisenda Julibert, unavailable in English. Barcelona, Plataforma Editorial, 2015.

A sword against vanity
Elias Canetti

Elias Canetti, a Jew of Sephardic origin, was born in Ruse, Bulgaria, in 1905. He studied in Vienna and was educated in the highest form of cosmopolitanism. Later he emigrated with his wife Veza Taubner-Calderón (1897-1963), also a writer, to London, the city where he lived, as well as Zurich, where he died in 1994. It was precisely his wife who introduced him to the play **Woyzeck**, by Georg Büchner (1813-1837), a book that changed his way of seeing the world as a writer. In 1981 he received the Nobel Prize for Literature.

Context: To speak of Canetti is to speak of Central Europe, of German as a powerful language, of a Jew who changes countries and whose homeland is language.

b. FRAGMENTS OF HIS WORK

> *"Grandiose words should whistle like a teapot, in which water is heated, as a warning."*

c. BRIEF COMMENTARY

Canetti's work analyses power and its devastating effect. He knows there is something shameful about winning, yet at the same time he knows that winning is surviving. This paradox identifies those lucid human beings who investigate the reasons and hollowness of every vain purpose.

No one has read more or thought better about society and power than this Nobel laureate. Canetti's stark lucidity surprises the reader with its enormous, extreme and characteristic viscerality of this key author of Central European Judaism.

d. EVERYDAY REFLECTIONS

Do not believe your own power. Do not get intoxicated by something that does not deserve posterity if it is not worth your effort. Analyse what is essential and live with a love that unites you to the earth, to people, to animals… It is with good reason that Canetti was fascinated by the animal kingdom.

Stop believing yourself to be an envoy of some almighty being and rid yourself of arrogance, which is nothing more than the ignorance that we are all humble, because *humility* comes from *humus*, the land from which we came and to which, without doubt, we will return.

Live life with ambition if you want – but always with respect – and seek humility. Look for tenderness within your core. Forget eternal commitments. It is often the path to perdition.

e. OTHER RELEVANT FRAGMENTS

"Act like you could never act again."

"I want to keep smashing myself until I am whole."

"Stop yourself before you say everything. Some say it all before beginning."

"No fool, no fanatic is ever going to take away the love of all those whose dreams have been overshadowed and cut short. Man will still become all things, the whole man. The slaves will free the masters."

"I would like to become tolerant without disregarding anything; not pursuing anyone, even if everyone was chasing me; to be better and better without realising it; be more and more sad, but to live at ease; to be more and more serene and cheerful, to be happy in others; not belonging to anyone, growing in everyone; loving the best, comforting the worst; I don't even hate myself anymore."

"You may have met three or four thousand people in your life, you will always speak of only six or seven."

"Living as if you had an entire lifetime. Meeting up with people every hundred years."

"The lowest man: the one to whom all his desires have been fulfilled."

"Big words should have to start whistling suddenly like those pots in which water is heated for tea, when it boils, they make it known."

"In any family other than your own, you suffocate.
You also suffocate in your own, but you don't notice."

"Since it became possible to obtain it by way of explosions,
Nothingness has lost its splendour and beauty."

"No man knows all the bitterness that awaits him, and if it
appeared suddenly, like a dream, he would reject it and look
away. This is what is called hope."

"The victor's state of satiety, his surfeit, his satisfaction, the
prolonged pleasure of his digestion. Some things would be
better if they didn't exist, but the only thing that should never
exist is a victor."

"But we are winners, of every man whom we know well and
who we survive. To win is to survive. How do you keep living
and still, however, not be a winner?"

f. SUGGESTED READING

The Human Province, New York, Farrar Straus & Giroux, 1986.
The Tongue Set Free, New York, Farrar Straus & Giroux, 1983.
The Conscience of Words New York, Farrar Straus & Giroux,
    1984.

He explained almost everything about the human condition

Anton Chekhov

a. WHO IS ANTON CHEKHOV?

Anton Pavlovich Chekhov (Taganrog, 1860 - Badenweiler, 1904), Russian doctor, storyteller and playwright and one of the greatest writers of all time. Grandson of Russian serfs, his grandfather, mujik, obtained freedom. His father, authoritarian, alcoholic and a devout Orthodox Christian, raised him fiercely. Chekhov put great effort into studying medicine in Moscow. In a letter of 1888 he wrote, "Medicine is my lawful wife, and literature is my mistress." His literary beginnings are humorous in tone, although in 1888, when already known to the public, he produced more profound writing in which he gave voice to the hard aspects of human existence.

A trip to the island of Sakhalin in 1890, made through Siberia on the way out and along the coasts of India on the way back, deeply marked his perspective, when he saw the conditions of the prisoners, an experience that he described as the "journey to hell". During the penury of 1892-1893 which hit southern Russia, Chekhov assisted in helping the starving. He then lived for a long period in the small estate of Melikhovo, not far from Moscow, where he wrote most of his work. He suffered from tuberculosis since 1887 and had to move to Crimea. From there he made frequent trips to France (Nice) and Germany as part of his treatment. The success of *The Seagull*, after being staged by Stanislavski, unexpectedly convinced Chekhov of his ability as a dramatic writer, after early doubts due to the initial failure of this same drama. The aforementioned work was followed, with great success, by *Uncle Vanya* in 1898-1899, *Three Sisters* in 1901 and *The Cherry Orchard* in 1904.

In 1901 he married actress Olga Knipper. He died in a German spa town and was transferred to Moscow on a refrigerated oyster train.

Context: What do we know about Tsarist Russia, that immense continent whose reality, undoubtedly so common and so different from ours, we can barely envisage? Who can teach us more about pain and *joie de vivre* than one of the greatest writers of all time? How much is Chekhov's depth owed to his triple status as a doctor, patient and genius? What does it mean to travel, at thirty years of age, already ill with tuberculosis, for eighty-two days by train to visit a prison, which he will write about and consider it to be hell? How transformed does he return from this hell? What is it to see hunger, pain and the essence of the human condition; an absolute desire for love, tenderness, shelter and affection?

Chekhov wrote, "The happier is my life, the darker are the stories I write," and at another time this genius of literature said, "I don't feel like writing; for the rest, it is difficult to unite the desire to live with the desire to write."

b. FRAGMENTS OF HIS WORK

"At Oreanda they sat on a seat not far from the church, looked down at the sea, and were silent. Yalta was hardly visible through the morning mist; white clouds stood motionless on the mountain-tops. The leaves did not stir on the trees, grasshoppers chirruped, and the monotonous hollow sound of the sea rising up from below, spoke of the peace, of the eternal sleep awaiting us. So it must have sounded when there was no Yalta, no Oreanda here; so it sounds now, and it will sound as indifferently and monotonously when we are all no more. And in this constancy, in this complete indifference to the life and death of each of us, there lies hid, perhaps, a pledge of our eternal salvation, of the unceasing movement of life upon earth, of unceasing progress towards perfection. Sitting beside a young woman who in the dawn seemed so lovely, soothed and spellbound in these magical surroundings—the sea, mountains, clouds, the open sky—Gurov thought how in reality everything is beautiful in this world when one reflects: everything except what we think or do ourselves when we forget our human dignity and the higher aims of our existence."

"A man walked up to them - probably a keeper - looked at them and walked away. And this detail seemed mysterious and beautiful, too. They saw a steamer come from Theodosia, with its lights out in the glow of dawn.

*'There is dew on the grass,' said Anna Sergeyevna, after a
silence.*

'Yes. It's time to go home.'

They went back to the town."

"He was tormented by an intense desire to confide his
memories to someone. But in his home it was impossible to
talk of his love, and he had no one outside; he could not talk
to his tenants nor to any one at the bank. And what had
he to talk of? Had he been in love, then? Had there been
anything beautiful, poetical, or edifying or simply interesting
in his relations with Anna Sergeyevna? And there was nothing
for him but to talk vaguely of love, of the woman, and no
one guessed what it meant; only his wife twitched her black
eyebrows, and said,

'The part of a lady-killer does not suit you at all, Dimitri.'"

"He explained that, too. He talked, thinking all the while
that he was going to see her, and no living soul knew of it, and
probably never would know. He had two lives: one, open, seen
and known by all who cared to know, full of relative truth and
of relative falsehood, exactly like the lives of his friends and
acquaintances; and another life running its course in secret.
And through some strange, perhaps accidental, conjunction of
circumstances, everything that was essential, of interest and of
value to him, everything in which he was sincere and did not
deceive himself, everything that made the kernel of his life,
was hidden from other people; and all that was false in him,
the sheath in which he hid himself to conceal the truth—
such, for instance, as his work in the bank, his discussions

at the club, his "lower race," his presence with his wife at anniversary festivities—all that was open. And he judged of others by himself, not believing in what he saw, and always believing that every man had his real, most interesting life under the cover of secrecy and under the cover of night. All personal life rested on secrecy, and possibly it was partly on that account that civilised man was so nervously anxious that personal privacy should be respected."

c. BRIEF COMMENTARY

Chekhov is the greatest short story writer of all time. His love for things, his very particular way of looking at and describing what is seemingly small are of an overwhelming intensity. He began to write with humour, and irony, but as the writer's work grew, his characters, all well-intentioned, proved themselves to be unskilled in the art of living; poorly equipped to face life. It is this clumsy, human helplessness that allowed us to relate to relate to them so well.

His story, ***The Lady with the Dog***, was made into a film in 1987. The film, directed by Nikita Mikhalkov and titled ***Dark Eyes***, featured a memorable Marcello Mastroianni, and Silvana Mangano, who filled both the screen and our lives with beauty and great nostalgia. In 1994, Louis Malle bowled us over with ***Vanya on 42ⁿᵈ Street***, where a group of actors, led by the wonderful Julianne Moore, rehearse ***Uncle Vanya***.

The famous commentary made by the great Russian author Vladimir Nabokov, who wrote some impressive reflections on the Chekhov's fine character, "Chekhov's intellectual was a man who combined the deepest human decency of which man is capable with an almost ridiculous inability to put his ideals and principles into action; a man devoted to moral beauty, the welfare of his people, the welfare of the universe, but unable in his private life to do anything useful; frittering away his provincial existence in a haze of utopian dreams; knowing exactly what is good, what is worthwhile living for, but at the same time sinking lower and lower in the mud of a humdrum existence, unhappy in love, hopelessly inefficient in everything - a good man who cannot make good. [...] He is unhappy, that man, and he makes others unhappy; he loves not his brethren, not those nearest to him, but the remotest. The plight of a negro in a distant land, of a Chinese coolie, of a workman in the remote Urals, affects him with a keener pang of moral pain than the misfortunes of his neighbour or the troubles of his wife. [...] Those men could dream; they could not rule. They broke their own lives and the lives of others, they were silly, weak, futile, hysterical..."

Raymond Carver wrote a beautiful story entitled **Errand**, dedicated to the Russian author's final days. Chekhov's list of admirers is impressive.

Life is a little greyer for those who have not discovered Chekhov, even if they do not know it. Because to read Chekhov is to know much, much more about how we humans are made.

d. EVERYDAY REFLECTIONS

The writer Simon Leys once famously said, that if you need to have surgery and have to choose between two surgeons of equal technical expertise, ensure you choose the one who has read Chekhov.

Why? Because undoubtedly between the two of them, whoever has discovered the stories of the Russian author and who has been moved by them, will most likely take much, much more than just the body of the patient to be operated on into consideration. The surgeon will know that there, on the operating table, is an entire life, the life of the patient, with their stories, their ties to others, their victories, joys, defeats and regrets. That surgeon will take care of a body and will be more aware of the great breadth of the word *life*.

How can Chekhov help us in real life?

I experienced the same situation, on the night of January 24, 2012 in room 505 of the Hotel de las Letras in Madrid.

That night, my wife told me on the phone that the next morning, urgently and without warning, they had to perform a test on my daughter Clara, who was five weeks old, to rule out cystic fibrosis. A terrible disease. There were no more trains or planes leaving for Barcelona.

I spent the night feeling distraught and very frightened.

Earlier I had read, at first silently and then aloud, a passage from Chekhov which is in room 505 (the excerpt from **The Lady and the Dog** shown on page 51).

Reading this kept me company. That night and the following morning, a father was waiting, distressed, in a quiet room, with Chekhov to keep him company. I felt very alone and read this beautiful text over and over again, and it did me a lot of good, even in a moment of such heartbreak.

In the morning, when, at 11:30 am they told me that everything was fine, I got down on my knees, in the middle of the room, and I wept with gratitude. In room 505. In the

Hotel de las Letras, number 11 Gran Vía street, Madrid.

Chekhov is the clearest proof that beauty is necessary to live, and that, beyond its apparent uselessness, it helps us to cope with life when there are clouds on the horizon, even when the storm does not come, but also when it does.

Reading Chekhov's stories is one of the greatest moments to experience the pleasure of reading, knowing that we are not alone.

e. OTHER RELEVANT FRAGMENTS

"Lord, don't allow me to condemn or to speak of what I do not know or do not understand."

"The torch of truth burns the hand which bears it."

"I have seen everything; however, now it is not about what I have seen, but how I have seen it."

"It is easier to write about Socrates than about a young woman or a cook."

"Don't try for too many characters. The centre of gravity should reside in two: he and she."

"A psychologist should not pretend to understand what he does not understand. Moreover, a psychologist should not convey the impression that he understands what no one understands. We shall not play the charlatan, and we will declare frankly that nothing is clear in this world. Only fools and charlatans know and understand everything."

"My holy of holies is the human body, health, intelligence, talent, inspiration, love, and absolute freedom—freedom from

violence and falsehood, no matter how the last two manifest themselves. This is the programme I would follow if I were a great artist."

f. SUGGESTED READING

The Essential Tales of Chekhov, Glasgow, Harper Perennial, 2000.
Ward No. 6 and Other Stories, London, Penguin Classics, 2002.
Cuentos completos ('Complete Stories'), unavailable in English.
Complete Plays, New York, WW Norton & Co., 2008.
How to Write Like Chekhov, New York, Hachette Book Group, 2016.

The union of the sacred and the human

Ralph Waldo Emerson

a. WHO IS RALPH WALDO EMERSON?

Ralph Waldo Emerson was an American writer, philosopher and poet. He was born in Boston in 1803 and died in Concord in 1882. He was the leader of the transcendentalist movement. His father was a minister in the Unitarian Church and his death, when Emerson was eight years old, left the family in complete poverty. Then, at fourteen years of age, he entered Harvard University.

The literary critic Harold Bloom said of him, "Emerson is not an easy read, but he was and remains the American sage, particularly in his great essay *Self-Reliance*. More than any other American – writer or not – Emerson captures the *ethos* of the American spirit. He knows what is uniquely American – individualism – and yet also provides continuity with general human aspirations throughout the ages. In a world that is becoming increasingly Americanized, we should all be reading Emerson."

Context: America is being formed. The enormous power and extraordinary energy of the most dynamic country of its time pivots on individualism and an infinite faith in the possibilities of effort.

b. FRAGMENTS OF HIS WORK

"Your dominion is as great as theirs, though without fine names. Build, therefore, your own world."

c. BRIEF COMMENTARY

What is most impressive about Emerson is that he says things which were before unheard of, that had been overlooked, that we dared not hear from ourselves. When you read them, however, it is as if your deepest convictions are being laid bare, those which had remained a secret because you did not have the courage to think, feel or say them.

If something touches you, Emerson seems to say, it is because it already existed within you.

d. EVERYDAY REFLECTIONS

Today's world is often overwhelming. It is easy to have doubts and doubt ourselves, even though we sometimes ride the arrogant horse of pride, to which Elias Canetti (1905-1994) alluded. Emerson immerses us in a powerful, humble, secret, peaceful and clear energy. He makes us grow in an undeniable way; this is why the author is constantly inviting us to be the masters of our own lives.

e. OTHER RELEVANT FRAGMENTS

"Give me health and a day, and I will make the pomp of emperors ridiculous. The dawn is my Assyria."

"Nothing is at last sacred but the integrity of your own mind."

"It is easy in the world to live after the world's opinion; it is easy in solitude to live after our own; but the great man is he who in the midst of the crowd keeps with perfect sweetness the independence of solitude."

"Insist on yourself. Never imitate."

"In general, every evil to which we do not succumb is a benefactor."

"Love and you shall be loved. All love is mathematically just, as much as the two sides of an algebraic equation."

"We reject affection and intimacy with people, as if we were waiting for greater affection and intimacy that are yet to come. But from where and when? Tomorrow will be like today. We waste life preparing to live."

"The one thing which we seek with insatiable desire is to forget ourselves, to be surprised out of our propriety, to lose our sempiternal memory and to do something without knowing how or why; in short to draw a new circle. Nothing great was ever achieved without enthusiasm. The way of life is wonderful; it is by abandonment."

"Never mind the ridicule, never mind the defeat: up again, old heart!"

"Before we acquire great power we must acquire wisdom to use it well."

"The man who renounces himself, comes to himself."

"He is rich who owns the day."

"Finish each day before you begin the next, and interpose a solid wall of sleep between the two. This you cannot do without temperance."

"One of the fundamental advantages of old age is the utter insignificance of achieving more or less success."

"For everything you gain, you lose something else."

f. SUGGESTED READING

Pensamientos para el futuro ('Thoughts for the Future'), unavailable in English. Barcelona, Península, 2002.
Self-Reliance, New York, ARC Manor, 2007.

Two thousand brilliant pages, like its elusive author

Elena Ferrante

a. WHO IS ELENA FERRANTE?

She was a great mystery, despite the enormous success of her incredible novels. Nothing was known about Elena Ferrante, a pseudonym behind which an extraordinary narrator was hidden, whose identity, apparently, only her editors knew. On the mystery of authorship, she herself said, "I don't regret my anonymity. As I see it, extracting the personality of the writer from the story he offers, from the characters he puts onstage, from the landscapes, from the objects, from interviews like this – in short, from the tonality of his writing entirely – is simply a good way of reading."* Finally, after an investigation by the newspaper *Il Sole 24 Ore*, on the hunt for the secret author, they followed the trail through searching for the enormous income that her royalties generated, and this led to uncovering the mystery: it was the translator Anita Raja, daughter of a Jewish family of Polish origin who fled the Holocaust and ended up in Naples.

Her **Neapolitan Novels** (which include **My Brilliant**

---

* Elena Ferrante in an email interview with Paolo di Stefano for Il Corriere della Sera.

Friend, **The Story of a New Name**, **Those Who Leave** and **Those Who Stay** and **The Story of a Lost Child**) have sold more than tens of thousands of copies in Spain.

Of all her books, the first of which was published in 1992, Elena Ferrante has sold 2.6 million copies in Italy, 1.6 million in the United States and Canada, and 600,000 in the United Kingdom. Rarely does this level of editorial quality go together with good sales. It seems it was only author Sandro Ferri, and Sandra Ozzola, both owners of the magnificent publishing house Edizioni e/o, and who publish the works of Elena Ferrante, among other fantastic titles, that knew the identity of the author. Whoever they are, we are dealing with books which are magnetic, hypnotic and truly joyous for those who read them.

Context: *L'amica geniale*, the original title of the first book of a tetralogy, published in 2011, is the beginning of a saga that re-enacts the lives of two women born in Naples, from their childhoods to their adult lives, and with it paints a great historical and social *fresco* from the 1950s to the present day.

Italy, the lives of two very close women, their families, their world, Naples, the post-war period, stories of various families that take us to the present day. All this. They are all powerful foundations on which to build this magnificent story.

If, in *War and Peace*, we lived through the Russia of the Napoleonic era, here we live, through the eyes of a woman, through post-war Italy and up to the present day, and we become a part of the lives of these few Neapolitan families with dazzling intensity.

Although the English edition of each book includes a

synopsis of the characters as a guide to remembering who is who, it is also helpful for browsing through the network of relationships between them. It is both a pleasant and demanding muddle, but it is worth it, like wading through the names of the protagonists of a Russian novel, their patronyms, diminutives, and so on.

There is no pleasure without surrender, nor anything that is worthwhile without effort.

b. FRAGMENTS OF HER WORK

"Their eyes were fixated on her… from Lila's moving body something had begun to emanate that they [the boys] noticed, an energy that stunned them, like the noise of beauty which was still to arrive, that was getting closer and closer." (**My Brilliant Friend**)

"Without love, it is not only the lives of people that dry up, but also those of the cities." (**My Brilliant Friend**)

"[…] she was among those who toiled day and night, who achieved magnificent results, who were treated with sympathy and appreciation, but who would never show off the high quality of those studies with the right attitude. I would always be afraid: afraid of saying the wrong thing, of using an exaggerated tone, of dressing unsuitably, of revealing petty feelings, of not having interesting thoughts." (**The Story of a New Name**)

c. BRIEF COMMENTARY

The 20th century has witnessed some of the most inspiring take-offs. I don't mean that of *Apollo 11* – no doubt remarkable – which, in 1969, reached the moon in four days, but that of women in all areas of life. Consciousness, taking off, the journey towards one's own emancipation and, in many cases, fulfilment. Whoever reads the ***Neapolitan Novels*** will discover why an author – and the world she describes – can take your breath away, reading four volumes that achieve something as colossal and admirable as conquering the moon. Reading Elena Ferrante is – whether you are a man or a woman – as wonderful, solid, splendid and unforgettable as two whole lives of two entire women can be. In the words of Juan Marsé, "Elena Ferrante's novels have kept me tied to my chair, reading and finding joy in pages where the emotion is never mundane."

We will not only talk about friendship, childhood, rivalries, growing up, boyfriends, the discovery of sex, love, pain, betrayal, secrets, ruptures, freedom, infidelities, family, work, studies, freedom... everything is here. All of it. And yet, there is one thread that seems to tie this masterpiece together: the value of education to provide emancipation, which is (entirely?) removed from the things that bind it: environment, family, the influence of the people you admire, love, hate and needs.

Yes, education as a way of building a person. The instruction that equips her with the extraordinary strength to escape the enormous force of gravity of her origins. Whoever reads this and has been the first in their family to have studied, will know how to recognise the material with which one of the two most extraordinary characters in this novel is made.

Canetti said something like, "all families are suffocating.

Your own family is too, you just don't realise it." This phrase from the Central European seems far from what the Southern Ferrante would say, but they are similar.

Both in the highly cultured family of Canetti, as you can read in his autobiography, and in the non-scholarly world of the characters in Elena Ferrante's novels, who muddle along and do what they can, in a certain way, they are both similar. In each world the protagonists are suffocated by their families. In the saga of the Italian Ferrante, the only character who frees herself from the severity of her world, in an indisputable way, although not absolute or definitive, is the one who knew how to create a unique destiny for herself through education.

Reading Elena Ferrante is to recharge the batteries of the pleasure of reading for a whole decade. Its protagonists will go with you throughout your life, like the characters in the films of Francis Ford Coppola and Sergio Leone, or like those of ***Rocco and His Brothers***, by Visconti.

d. EVERYDAY REFLECTIONS

He who writes this, has chosen Elena Ferrante out of infinite admiration. I have never learned anything about a familiar, extensive, yet at the same time intimate female world, in such a powerful and fascinating way. If in another chapter of this book I have chosen James Salter, it is because for me he is an author who explains a lot about a masculine way of feeling, defining a certain type of man.

Elena Ferrante explains the feminine register in a much broader way, with fascinating singularity. The ***Neapolitan Novels*** represent the cohort of many female worlds that demonstrate their admirable complexity, without wearing them down.

The sensation I felt of living inside the lives of two women and their worlds, and the admiration that I felt, throughout four extraordinary novels, took my breath away. I came out infinitely richer than when I went in.

Finally, I did not only learn about the female condition or how some women might think, feel and act. The novels are full of so many well drawn characters that it is within our power to feel totally or partially close to some of them or to certain moments in their lives.

A formidable literary work which is as formidable its protagonists.

e. OTHER RELEVANT FRAGMENTS

"'Nothing.'

'The revolution, the workers, the new world, and that other bullshit?'

'Stop it. If you've unexpectedly decided to make a truthful speech I'm listening, otherwise let's forget it.'

'May I point out something? You always use true and truthfully, when you speak and when you write. Or you say: "unexpectedly". But when do people ever speak truthfully and when do things ever happen unexpectedly? You know better than I that it's all a fraud and that one thing follows another and then another. I don't do anything truthfully anymore, Lenù. And I've learned to pay attention to things. Only idiots believe that they happen unexpectedly.'

'Bravo. What do you want me to believe, that you have

everything under control, that it's you…'"

"In stories you do what you want and in real life you do what you can."

"On the other hand, in those days in France I felt I was in the center of chaos and, nevertheless, endowed with instruments to recognize its laws."

"It didn't take long for me to discover that I was getting used to feeling happy and unhappy at the same time, as if that were the inevitable state of my life."

"In what disorder we lived, how many fragments of ourselves were scattered, as if to live were to explode into splinters."

f. SUGGESTED READING

The four volumes of the Neapolitan Novels are:

My Brilliant Friend, London, Europa Editions, 2012.
The Story of a New Name, London, Europa Editions, 2013.
Those Who Leave and Those Who Stay, London, Europa
     Editions, 2013.
The Story of a Lost Child, London, Europa Editions, 2015.

The meaning (of life) is a choice

Viktor Frankl

a. WHO IS VIKTOR FRANKL?

Viktor E. Frankl (Vienna, 1905-1997), Austrian neurologist and psychiatrist from a Jewish family, is the founder of logotherapy. Influenced in his early days by Freud and Adler, he later distanced himself from their teachings. After surviving as a prisoner in various Nazi concentration camps (including Auschwitz and Dachau), a tragic time in which he lost his wife and most of his family, he carried out his teaching work at various universities, such as Vienna, Harvard and Stanford, and gave numerous lectures around the world. He received twenty-nine honorary doctorates.

He is the author of more than thirty books, of which tens of millions of copies have been sold and they have been translated into numerous languages. His principal work, **Man's Search for Meaning**, is one of the ten most influential texts in the US according to a survey by the United States Library of Congress.

Context: Let's put Judaism, Nazism and a prisoner, yet still a free man, all together. Let's imagine that absolute horror is brought face to face with the willingness for meaning. Let's imagine that absolute evil goes up against the absolute force of the individual, who is nevertheless alone and free to decide.

And let's see who wins, who destroys (or overcomes) whom.

b. FRAGMENTS OF HIS WORK

"I remember two cases of would-be suicide. Which bore a striking similarity to each other. Both men had talked of their intentions to commit suicide. Both used the typical argument—they had nothing more to expect from life. In both cases it was a question of getting them to realize that life was still expecting something from them; something in the future was expected of them. We found, in fact, that for the one it was his child whom he adored and who was waiting for him in a foreign country. For the other it was a thing. Not a person. This man was a scientist and had written a series of books which still needed to be finished. His work could not be done by anyone else, any more than another person could ever take the place of the father in his child's affections.

This uniqueness and singleness which distinguishes each individual and gives a meaning to his existence has a bearing on creative work as much as it does on human love. When the impossibility of replacing a person is realized, it allows the responsibility which a man has for his existence and its continuance to appear in all its magnitude. A man who becomes conscious of the responsibility he bears toward a human being who affectionately waits for him, or to an unfinished work, will never be able to throw away his life. He knows the 'why' for his existence, and will be able to bear almost any 'how.'"

"From all this we may learn that there are two races of men in this world, but only these two — the "race" of the decent man and the "race" of the indecent man. Both are found everywhere; they penetrate into all groups of society. No group consists entirely of decent or indecent people.

Life in a concentration camp tore open the human soul and exposed its depths.

Is it surprising that in those depths we again found only human qualities which in their very nature were a mixture of good and evil? The rift dividing good from evil, which goes through all human beings, reaches into the lowest depths and becomes apparent even on the bottom of the abyss which is laid open by the concentration camp.

We have come to know him as perhaps no generation before us has; What then is man? Man is that being which invented the gas chambers; but he is at the same time that being which walked with head held high into these very same gas chambers, the Lord's Prayer or the Jewish prayer for the dead on his lips."

c. BRIEF COMMENTARY

When some texts are as powerful and clear as the *Man's Search for Meaning*, commenting on them could lead to ridicule. Frankl must be read from a perspective of absolute humility. In silence. And then spoken to about his questions and propositions.

Here, however, we will venture to say that the search for truth, the desire for a clean and honourable perspective, even after almost being destroyed, has the redemptive power of the human condition.

When, in the middle of the night, when you are going through difficulty or doubt, and everything around you is collapsing, clinging on to Viktor Frankl is a unique opportunity to save yourself.

d. EVERYDAY REFLECTIONS

The question about good and evil, about decent and indecent, about freedom of action, what it costs, and its consequences, is an opportunity to call the trivial, trivial, and to disarm it. And to put into hierarchical order what is important in life.

Frankl practises, among many other things, a generosity of forgiveness. Furthermore, he gives us the courage to remind ourselves of the role of responsibility, since it was he who proposed, for the first time, that a Statue of Responsibility be erected on the west coast of the United States, to complete and supplement that of Liberty.

e. OTHER RELEVANT FRAGMENTS

"Contrary to energy sources, meaning is inexhaustible."

f. SUGGESTED READING

Man's Search for Meaning, Boston, Beacon Press, 2006.
Viktor E. Frankl. El sentido de la vida, de Elisabeth Lukas, Barcelona, Plataforma Editorial, 2008.
... Yes to Life: In Spite of Everything, Boston, Beacon Press, 2020.

Our own wings
André Gide

a. WHO IS ANDRÉ GIDE?

Born in Paris in 1869, André Gide, the son of a law professor at the University of Paris, grew up in Normandy. He suffered from health problems during his childhood and was solitary in nature. He married his cousin in 1895, but they never consummated the relationship. Years later, in 1924, he received harsh criticism after publishing *Corydon*, a work in which he defended homosexuality. He had an enormous influence on various authors, including Albert Camus (1913-1960), and received the Nobel Prize for Literature in 1947. He died in his native Paris in 1951.

Context: Gide lived in France's colonial heyday and denounced the actions of his country after travelling to Africa with his lover, the Swiss film director Marc Allégret (1900-1973).

He was rejected by several of his friends after the publication of his book Return from the USSR (1936), where he denounced the situation of the Soviet Union after his trip to the communist country.

This double tension, both personal and national, led him to work through ethical and moral issues with great determination.

b. FRAGMENTS OF HIS WORK

"And now, Nathaniel, throw away my book. Shake yourself free of it. Leave me. Leave me; now you are in my way; you hamper me; I have exaggerated my love for you and it occupies me too much. I am tired of pretending I can educate anyone. When have I said that I wanted you to be like me? It is because you differ from me that I love you; the only thing I love in you is what differs from me. Educate! Whom should I educate but myself? Yes, Nathaniel, I have educated my self interminably. And I have not done yet. I only esteem myself for my possibilities.

Nathaniel, throw away my book; do not let it satisfy you. Do not think your truth can be found by anyone else; be ashamed of nothing more than of that. If I found your food for you, you would have no appetite for it; if I made your bed, you would not be able to sleep in it.

Throw away my book; say to yourself that it is only one of the thousand possible postures in life. Look for your own. Do not do what someone else could do as well as you. Do not say, do not write what someone else could say, could write as well as you. Care for nothing in yourself but what you feel exists nowhere else, and out of yourself create, impatiently or patiently, ah! the most irreplaceable of beings."

c. BRIEF COMMENTARY

This text has a foundational force. The energy it transmits, the beauty and delicacy it displays are like the text of a personal constitution that every human being has the right (and duty) to build.

There are few texts which are so beautiful. You would need to look at Walt Whitman (1819-1892) to find lines of similar breathtaking quality.

d. EVERYDAY REFLECTIONS

Many people wait for some kind of biological, social or economic imperative to have their mid-life crisis. But many people could avoid it (completely, or at least minimise its intensity) if they immersed themselves in Gide's teachings.

Gide doesn't give us permission to be ourselves: he demands it. How many things have we missed through playing a role that was imposed on us by others!

Let us celebrate our own authenticity and make Pindar's exhortation (6th century BC) come true:

"May learning make you who you are."

e. OTHER RELEVANT FRAGMENTS

"No evolutionist could assume that there was any relationship between the caterpillar and the butterfly if it were not known that they are precisely the same being. Affiliation seems impossible and there is identity. I think that if I had been a naturalist, I would have directed all the forces and all the questions of my spirit towards that enigma."

"'Know thyself'. A maxim is as pernicious as it is ugly. 'Whoever studies himself' arrests his own development. A caterpillar who seeks to know himself would never become a butterfly."

"I clearly feel a constancy through my diversity; what I feel to be diverse is always me. But precisely because I know and I feel that this constancy exists, why try to obtain it?"

f. SUGGESTED READING

The Counterfeiters, London, Penguin Classics, 1990.
The Fruits of the Earth, London, Vintage Classics, 2002.
Journals, vol. 1, Illinois, University of Illinois Press, 2000.

When childhood is your strength
Natalia Ginzburg

a. WHO IS NATALIA GINZBURG?

Natalia Ginzburg (Palermo, 1916 - Rome, 1991) is one of the greatest writers of the 20th century. She came from an educated family and spent most of her life between Turin and Rome. Her father, of Jewish origin, was a professor of medicine, and her mother, a Catholic, was the daughter of a socialist lawyer. She grew up in a liberal and artistic environment. She wrote plays, essays and narratives and won awards such as the Viareggio, the Tempo and the Strega. Political commitment marked her life and work. She married the Jewish intellectual Leone Ginzburg, who was assassinated in 1943 by the fascist regime. She was co-founder of Einaudi, one of the key publishing houses of 20th century Europe, and worked with Giulio Einaudi, Cesare Pavese, Massimo Mila and Italo Calvino. She was a deputy for the Italian Communist Party. She translated Proust, Flaubert and Maupassant.

Context: To speak of Natalia Ginzburg is to speak of a cultured, emancipated, committed woman, and a pioneer of the so-called "feminine literature". It is also to touch on a work described by Italo Calvino as quintessentially beautiful and deeply sad, and to read someone who described family relationships in a way that only one other Italian author, Elena Ferrante, was able to do so masterfully many years later.

Italy has always been the scene of great beauty, but in the 20th century it was also the setting for two terrible wars and movements of very strong commitment and resistance, and this magnificent author speaks of it all. Reading Natalia Ginzburg is a tremendous discovery.

b. FRAGMENTS OF HER WORK

"I shall look at the clock and keep track of the hours, vigilant and attentive to everything, I shall take care that my children's feet are always warm and dry, at least during infancy. And perhaps, for learning to walk in worn-out shoes, it is as well to have dry, warm feet when we are children."

c. BRIEF COMMENTARY

Childhood is seldom discussed among adults and if it is, it is mentioned briefly and with embarrassment; even more so among those people who have been marked by success. Whether it is for the sake of discretion in the presence of this sacred space (when it is), fear, this aforementioned embarrassment, prudence, or even - let's hope not - by having forgotten the only space where some lucky people have known happiness.

However, on some occasions, even those who have not had a happy childhood have spoken and written about it with tenderness and luminosity. There are also those who have known an intellectually rich, powerful and full life and seem to ignore childhood. For a false appearance of strength, or for other reasons.

The relationship of a human being with their own childhood is the most beautiful, complex and ignored territory, most of the time. This is not the case of Natalia Ginzburg, whose story **"Worn out shoes"**, written within the magnificent work *The Little Virtues*, is like a compendium of this writer's human generosity.

d. EVERYDAY REFLECTIONS

There is greatness in the lucidity of Natalia Ginzburg. There is a will for clarity and truth. There is enormous courage in her destiny and a demanding, graceful and relentless serenity.

Her perspective is, in the words of Carmen Martín Gaite, who writes a beautiful prologue entitled "El látigo de la vocación" ('The whip of vocation') for *All Our Yesterdays*, that of someone who "allowed a filtering of the piety, bewilderment and greatness of humble beings who suffer from a cruel fate without understanding it, like random wind blades."

Giving *The Little Virtues* as a gift is one of the best things one can do in caring for a sensitive friend.

e. OTHER RELEVANT FRAGMENTS

"When I'm doing anything else, when I study a foreign language, try to learn typing or geography, or try to speak in public or knit or travel, I suffer: I keep asking myself how other people manage to do these things…, I seem to be deaf and blind and I feel a sort of nausea deep inside me. When

I'm writing though, I never think there might be a better way, to which other writers resort. I'm not concerned at all about how other writers go about it… That is my job and I will work at it until I die. I'm very content with that work and I wouldn't change it for anything in the world. I realised it was my job a long time ago. Between the ages of five and ten I still had my doubts about it, and rather fancied myself as a painter or conquering countries on horseback, or inventing some sort of important new machine. But from the time I was ten I always knew it… Besides, I couldn't even imagine my life without this taskmaster. He has always been there, has never left me even for a moment; and when I thought he was asleep, his watchful, shining gaze was still upon me.

That is how my job is. As for money - well, it doesn't bring me much, and so I always have to have other work at the same time to live on. Yet at times it does pay a bit, and to have money from this source is a very pleasant thing, like receiving money and presents from a lover."

"This job is a stern master, a master capable of whipping us until we bleed, a boss who blames us and yells at us. We have to swallow saliva and tears and grit our teeth and dry our bleeding wounds and serve him. Serve him when he asks it. Then he helps us stand up and keep our feet firmly on the ground. He helps us conquer madness and delirium, desperation and fever. But he must give the orders, and when we need him he always refuses to pay attention to us… It is a job that feeds on the best and worst of our life; our bad feelings as well as our good ones flow in its bloodstream. It feeds on us and grows in us."

"He used to say that he knew his art so thoroughly that it was impossible he should discover any further secret in it, and because it could not promise him any more secrets it no longer interested him. We felt humiliated by the fact that we bored him, but we were unable to tell him that we saw only too clearly where his mistake lay - in his refusal to love the daily current of existence, which flows on freely and apparently without secrets… He died in the summer. In summer our city is deserted and seems very large, clear and echoing, like an empty city square; the sky has a milky pallor… None of us were there. He chose to die on an ordinary, stifling hot day in August, and he chose a room in a hotel near the station.

He wanted to die like a stranger in the city to which he belonged."

f. SUGGESTED READING

All Our Yesterdays, New York, Skyhorse Publishing, 2015.
A Family Lexicon, London, Daunt Books, 2018.
Dear Michael, London, Peter Owen Publishers, 1974.
The Little Virtues, London, Daunt Books, 2018.

The tenderness of a hard heart

Patricia Highsmith

a. WHO IS PATRICIA HIGHSMITH?

The life of Patricia Highsmith (Forth Worth, Texas, 1921-Locarno, 1995) was marked by her voracity for reading from a young age, which she was able to do thanks to her mother and stepfather's extensive library, where, at the age of eight, she came across and read Karl Menninger's book ***The Human Mind***, and it left her fascinated by the subject of mental disorders. Her passion for writing was a constant throughout the years: she began to write when she was very young, she kept a diary all her life and wrote more than twenty novels, as well as stories for children and some writing manuals. She had an intense, unresolved, love-hate relationship with her mother, who confessed, according to her own account, that she had tried to abort her daughter during pregnancy by drinking turpentine.

She was considered by some to be harsh, cruel, unfriendly and misogynistic, and by others as simply dry, of few words, but funny. Undoubtedly, she was someone exceptional. She was a lesbian and it seems that it was difficult for her to maintain lasting and stable relationships.

She rewrote her first novel, **_Strangers on a Train_**, on the advice of Truman Capote and published it in 1950, with relative success; however, the 1951 film adaptation by Hitchcock greatly increased her reputation. She was soon known for her irony, harsh prose, and disturbing, amoral characters, who were mostly young, attractive, and emotionally unstable men. Her reading creates an addiction.

As the bookseller Regina says in her blog _Regina Exlibris_: "Highsmith takes you hurtling down the tracks of her plots, which are at times vertiginous and at times lethargic. She dissects psychopathy and passes it on to you. She takes away your empathy with the victims, and she takes you to the limits of suspicion and paranoia, and portrays human stupidity – yours included. To round it off, there is no domestic paradise that does not poison, nor atmosphere that does not cloud over. Her fiction is not police, crime or detective; it is suspense. In her stories there are plots, crimes and victims, but there are no heroes or seedy alleyways. She immerses you in highly-charged ecosystems where suspicion envelops you like a viscous mass that you cannot get rid of. You are trapped together with a character and surrounded by police, by debt collectors, by her obsessions and by who knows what else."

Context: Although American, Highsmith lived much of her life in Europe. She believed in American democratic ideals, but was also very critical of the reality of her country's culture and foreign policy, where she was labelled an anti-Semite for having supported the cause of the liberation of Palestine, even though she had close friends who were Jews, like Arthur Koestler.

Highsmith was, as mentioned before, a lesbian. Although she knew that her sexuality could never been seen in a positive in New York in the early 1950s, she nevertheless launched herself into describing her great love.

She wrote the plot of her novel ***Carol*** in one go, over the course of one night, after a chance encounter with a woman who left her thunderstruck. This meeting took place in a department store in New York, where Patricia eventually worked as a shop assistant.

At that time, the book was called ***The Price of Salt*** and published under a pseudonym, in order to hide what I seem to recall Marguerite Yourcenar describing as "a certain way of loving."

The book, a high point in the writer's career, was considerably mature for a young author of barely thirty years of age. It tells a story of seduction, suspense, acceptance and love, and was hugely successful, most likely due to its happy ending, which was very unusual at the time.

Thirty-eight years later, in 1989, she reprinted with a different title: ***Carol***. She signed it with her own name and revealed the understandable reasons for her initial anonymity. She also said, "I'm glad to think that this book gave thousands of lonely and scared people something to lean on."

It's funny to think that the money she earned as a shop assistant at that time was used to pay for the psychoanalysis treatment that led her to take the decision not to marry the boyfriend she was going out with.

b. FRAGMENTS OF HER WORK

"It would be almost like love, what she felt for Carol, except that Carol was a woman. It was not quite insanity, but it was certainly blissful."

"'What could be duller than past history!'
'Maybe futures that won't have any history.'"

"I feel I stand in a desert with my hands outstretched, and you are raining down upon me."

"I think friendships are the result of certain needs that can be completely hidden from both people, sometimes hidden forever."

"The dusky and faintly sweet smell of her perfume came to Therese again, a smell suggestive of dark-green silk, that was hers alone, like the smell of a special flower."

"Was life, were human relations like this always, Therese wondered. Never solid ground underfoot. Always like gravel, a little yielding, noisy so the whole world could hear, so one always listened, too, for the loud, harsh step of the intruder's foot."

"Then Carol slipped her arm under her neck, and all the length of their bodies touched fitting as if something had prearranged it. Happiness was like a green vine spreading through her, stretching fine tendrils, bearing flowers through her flesh. She had a vision of a pale white flower, shimmering as if seen in darkness, or through water. Why did people talk of heaven, she wondered."

"She remembered the detective's face and the barely legible expression that she realized now was malice. It was malice

she had seen in his smile, even as he said he was on no side, and she could feel in him a desire that was actually personal to separate them, because he knew they were together. She had seen just now what she had only sensed before, that the whole world was ready to be their enemy, and suddenly what she and Carol had together seemed no longer love or anything happy but a monster between them, with each of them caught in a fist."

"But the most important point I did not mention and was not thought of by anyone - that is rapport between two men and two women can be absolute and perfect, as it can never be between man and woman, and perhaps some people want just this, as others want that more shifting and uncertain things that happens between men and women. It was said of at least implied yesterday that my present course would bring me to the depths of human vice and degeneration. Yes, I have sunk a good deal since they took you from me. It is true, if I were to go on like this and be spied upon, attacked, never possessing one person long enough so that knowledge of a person is a superficial thing- that is degeneration. Or to live against one's grain, that is degeneration by definition."

c. BRIEF COMMENTARY

Carol left me speechless when I read it. It is mesmerising. Without a hint of melodrama or tragedy, she describes her love, in an almost naive, very natural way.

There are no rough sex scenes, there are no regrets, she picks through emotions and moods with great precision and great delicacy. I had never read such a seemingly easy and natural text which was about something seemingly so out of the ordinary.

With determination and courage, Highsmith sets out to talk about a relationship between women. However, she does it so well, that it ends up being about the fragility of any relationship; in a way it becomes a book about insecurity during the fragile and euphoric period of falling in love, when the full range of emotions is condensed into milliseconds.

She is always restrained, corrosive, without excesses and not at all sanctimonious. She knows exactly how to gauge the level of tenderness, she does not renounce her sharp and perverse humour. She leaves us with interesting reflections, and she gives us details of a certain depth, with tantalising dialogue.

d. EVERYDAY REFLECTIONS

In North American narrative there is a continuity of authors (who come one after the other, from the works of Katherine Anne Porter to Raymond Carver) who have described the human need for love, tenderness and solidarity in environments whose massification and opulence show our vulnerability in a much more obvious way. How fantastic are these Americans when they talk about love!

Highsmith is part of this club. She appeals to our intelligence and our feelings to make us understand and highlight the extraordinary part of any habitual emotion, at the same time as knowing how to deal with extraordinary situations, narrating them in such a way that they appear much closer to us.

For her, the most common and boring routines are full of possibilities and surprises, and the most explosive and surprising feelings are part of the most common reality. Her vision enriches our daily life.

e. OTHER RELEVANT FRAGMENTS

> *"Carol was beautiful and Therese did not understand why her days had to be so empty if she was made to live with people who loved her, walking through a beautiful house or through beautiful cities or along blue coasts with a great horizon and a blue sky in the background."*

> *"I want the sun throbbing on my head like chords of music. I think of a sun like Beethoven, a wind like Debussy, and birdcalls like Stravinsky. But the tempo is all mine."*

f. SUGGESTED READING

Carol, London, Bloomsbury Publishing, 2010.
Strangers on a Train, London, Vintage Publishing, 1999.
The Talented Mr. Ripley, London, Virago Press, 2020.

The finest journalism
of the 20th century
Ryszard Kapuscinski

Ryszard Kapuscinski was born in Poland, in 1932, in Pinsk
(now in Belarus), and he died in Warsaw in 2007. He studied
History at the University of Warsaw and devoted his life to
journalism. He contributed to *Time, The New York Times, La
Jornada* and *Frankfurter Allgemeine Zeitung*. Since 1962 he
combined his journalistic work with literary activity and was
professor at several universities. Between 1954 and 1981 he
was a member of the Polish Communist Party. In 1964 he
was appointed by the Polish Press Agency as its only foreign
correspondent, a profession he fulfilled until 1981. He
travelled through developing countries and reported on wars,
coups and revolutions in Asia, Europe and Latin America.
He was perhaps the best-known journalist working on the
African continent in the 1960s and 1970s, when he witnessed
first-hand the end of the European colonial empires.

Among the awards and distinctions he received, the
following should be highlighted: the 2003 Prince of Asturias
Award for Communication and Humanities; and receiving
an honorary doctorate from the University of Krakow, the

University of Gdansk, the University of Silesia in Katowice, the University of Wroclaw, the University of Barcelona and the University Ramon Llull. He also received the Elsa Morante Letterario Prize (2005) and was a member of the European Academy of Sciences and Arts.

Context: It cannot have been easy to be born and raised in Poland in 1932, a country between Germany and Russia in the 20th century. Not only the two great blocs, East and West, but also the so-called "Third World" were paraded before Ryszard Kapuscinski alternative vision. He was a curious and honest journalist, who retold the world with depth and lucidity.

To read him is like incorporating the lives of poor people in poor countries into our own. People we cannot forget, the challenges of living (and surviving) in empires, the situations which create the world's important political conflicts. Life and death. Exclusion and power. Glory and anonymity. The security and fear of the hand of cards that history holds for each human being, marked by where, and in what time and environment, they were born.

He writes in a unique way, with empathy, simplicity, humility and an extraordinary capacity for understanding. It is with good reason that his work has been translated into dozens of languages. He is the greatest journalist of the 20th century.

b. FRAGMENTS OF HIS WORK

"In the Third World you have to have one of two things: either time or money. It is an iron principle of the job of a reporter. He who does not have time but has large sums to spend can

achieve whatever he sets his mind to. He who has no money
but has time to spare can also get everything he wants."

"If we refuse to know the other, we can enter a tragic stage,
of great conflicts, of death. In war I have learned one thing:
when prisoners are taken and the soldiers from the opposing
side are interrogated, always, always, always, the same pattern
is repeated, the same model: the soldier has been prepared to
ignore everything about his enemy. The enemy, the other, is
abstract for him. And the moment he starts to know the other,
he starts talking, he loses his motivation for the fight."

"Requirements for being a reporter: have good health, mental
resistance, curiosity for the world, know foreign languages;
knowing how to travel, being open to other people and other
cultures, feeling passion for the job and, finally, trying to pass
it all through the sieve of reflection."

"When I am among the nomads of the Sahara, I show them
all my respect, because if I, without knowing their culture
and without that knowledge that allows them to survive, were
to find myself in their place, I would simply have died. All
European civilisation would be of little or nothing to me…
The mere struggle to preserve life in those conditions is a
superhuman effort. It is not, of course, productive knowledge:
it does not serve to create a new generation of computers or to
make great scientific discoveries.
But they are no less worthy of respect for that."

"War is a disaster, always… I remember when Africa or
Asia still had a great inferiority complex towards the West,
a tremendous humility. Now things have changed! When you

travel the world you discover numerous civilisations who are proud of their identity, Islam, Hinduism, the indigenous Latin Americans, the Chinese. All of them are ready to defend their identity, to underline their own values. They ask for a place at the great table of the world, to which they also belong."

c. BRIEF COMMENTARY

To read Kapuscinski is to surrender to the privilege of looking at and understanding the world. It is the joy of traveling with the mind. It is being in the middle of history. It is feeling that learning is a constant privilege. It is understanding things that no one has ever said before. Kapuscinski has the most amazing vision. He is the closest reflection. He has the humility of not judging. He is the smile that seeks to understand. There are few occasions when the writer of this book has been happier reading something. Meeting him also increased my admiration for this character. Humble, endearing, deep, curious, kind and funny.

I have been reading Kapuscinski for forty years now, and, along with Camus, he is the author of whom I have enjoyed more works than any other. Reading Kapuscinski is a very powerful vaccine against fear of the other, against the unknown. Nobody teaches you how to see so clearly. There is no way back after looking at the world through the eyes of this genius. An almost perfect secondary school education could be achieved through a calm, reasoned and argued reading of *A Reporter's Self Portrait*.

Reading Kapuscinski is to enjoy pure freedom.

d. EVERYDAY REFLECTIONS

Today we read newspapers often to be poisoned by reality. Learning about the news is often intoxicating, told in its usual way, in the context in which we live. This knowledge, and the way it is told to us, makes us who we are. Not only our opinion, but our way of living and responding, of doing, deciding and thinking. It is certainly more brutal not to read them, although through avoiding the brutality of ignorance, we fall into the toxicity of "the news," as it is chosen, cut out and interpreted for us. Only the immense vision of someone who can overcome this information using their own judgement can encourage us to look at the world with empathy, with depth of field, with generous intensity, with curiosity that redeems indifference.

Reading Kapuscinski is to brighten your gaze, to give it hope, even when what he is describing is so severe. I don't know through what mechanism, but reading it is exhilarating, it is restorative. It is to humanise travel. It is to enter into the other. It is the gift of the only impossible journey: that of the humble discovery of the greatness of this world, which we can never understand without knowing how to look, without knowing how to think.

e. OTHER RELEVANT FRAGMENTS

"What difference does it make if they say 16 roubles or 18 roubles? It is a detail that holds no importance; the important thing is that they are poor, so very poor."

"... No, it is not a global village we live in, but a global train or underground station, through which the swarm of David Riesman's "lonely crowd" passes, made up of busy, stressed-out people, who are indifferent towards each other and who do not want to be approached to be in proximity with another. In fact, it seems that the more electronic devices we have, the less connection and human contact there is."

"The process of globalisation and creation of the planetary society is irreversible. So one of two: either we start to hate, fight, disregard and perceive the other as the enemy... or we start to seek mutual understanding and knowledge. 99% of the conflicts that shake the world are born out of ignorance!"

"Because war never starts with the first shot. War begins with a change of language."

f. SUGGESTED READING

Shah of Shahs, London, Penguin Classics, 2006.
El mundo de hoy ('The World of Today'), unavailable in English.
Imperium, London, Granta Books, 2019.
The Shadow of the Sun, London, Penguin, 2002.
Il cinico non è adatto a questo mestiere ('A Cynic Wouldn't Suit This Profession'), unavailable in English.

Let time build solid castles with what looked like sand

Hiromi Kawakami

a. WHO IS HIROMI KAWAKAMI?

Hiromi Kawakami is one of the most popular current Japanese writers in her country, and one of the most awarded and celebrated in the entire world. She was born in 1958 in Tokyo and studied Natural Sciences at Ochanomizu Women's University, graduating in 1980 with her work on sea urchins. She wrote and worked for a science fiction magazine, *NW-SF*, where she had her first story published. She also taught biology for a time at a secondary school, until she had to leave to go with her husband, who was forced to move for work. She then made her family a priority for a few years.

In 1994, at the age of thirty-six, Kawakami made her debut as a literary fiction writer, with a book of short stories titled **Kamisama** ('God'). In 1996 she won one of Japan's most prestigious literary awards, the Akutagawa, for her work **Hebi wo fumu** ('Strange Weather in Tokyo').

Since then she has won the most prestigious awards in Japan and her novels have crossed borders and been translated into numerous languages.

Context: Kawakami studied at a women's university, worked as a teacher in an institute, got married, had children, left her job to follow her husband to another city for work…

It sounds like the story of a conventional woman in a very conventional Japan, and yet she harbours exceptional literary ability and an unusual delicacy.

As François Simon says: "Her words pass like a warm breeze through the mosquito net. There exists in them the enchantment of a song."

There is also the committed Kawakami, who reacted with clarity after the tragedy suffered by Japan in 2011, when there was an earthquake followed by a tsunami, and which severely affected much of the country. Due to its great relevance, we have partially reproduced a long text. Kawakami says,

"Unless you live in this country, it is difficult to take charge, but it is true that Japanese people live in fear of a violent earthquake, yet at the same time they are willing to deal with it.

Everything leads us to believe that the feeling of impermanence that permeates the Japanese people comes precisely from the beauty that nature has given this country. He who benefits from nature must face its cruelty no matter what. Nature bestows without saying anything and, in the same way, starts without hesitation. The human being is powerless before this law from which they cannot escape. Even the inhabitants of the big cities feel the contradiction between the extraordinary goodness of nature and its inclemency.

[…] Life is instability. This philosophy of impermanence is the basis of the behaviour of those who help each other in silence. Yes, life is synonymous with impermanence, yes, the

human being is ephemeral, yes, everyone is alone when they are born, alone when they die and, precisely for this reason, we must help each other to save ourselves. […] I am nothing more than an insignificant thing. A sad observation perhaps. But that is exactly what makes my life precious. […]

Knocked down by typhoons, crushed by earthquakes, we have lived for a thousand years, two thousand years. And while life is here, we become aware of luminous moments which do not have a number. The beauty of the twilight. The magic of cherry blossom petals blown away by the wind. The inestimable value of the neighbour that we suddenly perceive, for something which is nothing. The pleasure of a sunset in the company of friends. The pleasures evoked by the ending of the day, in that moment that precedes the dream. In my insignificance, I know very well that these seconds will never know eternity and that this is precisely what makes them shine in my eyes with an ever more vivid radiance. This twinkle is precious, and unequalled. I feel love for this glow that fades as soon as it is born. It gives me joy. It saddens me, too. I believe that it is this brief glow that I try to capture and introduce in my novels.

[…] If it is an earthquake or a tsunami, I believe that the Japanese people will resign themselves to the misfortune. But the same will not happen with regard to the accident at the nuclear power plant, which is still in a critical condition at the time of writing this, on 25 March 2011, and a resignation or acceptance of the situation is out of the question for me."

b. FRAGMENTS OF HER WORK

"I was looking at the sky. I had sat down on a large log. Toru, Satoru and the teacher had disappeared into the forest. From where I stood, the hammering of the woodpecker was almost inaudible. Other birds chirped in its place [...]. Small blue patches were visible among the treetops. The foliage looked like a web stretched across the sky. When my eyes adjusted to the darkness, I detected many forms of life in the undergrowth: moss, small orange mushrooms [...]. I saw dead beetles, infinite varieties of ants, insects of all kinds, and butterflies that slept on the undersides of the leaves.

I was surprised to be surrounded by so many living creatures. In the city I was always alone, even if I was with the teacher. I thought that only large creatures lived in cities. However, reflecting on the matter, I realised that in the city I was also surrounded by living beings. We were never alone. Although in the tavern I only spoke to the teacher. Satoru was there as well as a crowd of regulars whose faces looked familiar to me. Still, I had never considered other people to be of flesh and blood. I hadn't realised that each one of them had their own life, full of ups and downs like mine."

"I would like to talk about the only time the teacher called me from his mobile phone. I knew he was calling me from his mobile because of the background noise I could hear on the other end of the line.

'Tsukiko,' he said.
'Yes.'
'Tsukiko.'
'Yes.'"

"On that occasion it was I who answered in monosyllables, as if we had exchanged roles.

'You are a sweetheart, Tsukiko.'

'What?'

That was all I said before suddenly hanging up. I called him right away, but he didn't answer. After two hours I called him back on the landline. He picked up the phone and answered calmly, as if nothing had happened."

c. BRIEF COMMENTARY

Kawakami writes with delicacy, subtlety, tenderness and depth. In **Strange Weather in Tokyo**, a thirty-eight-year-old woman, Tsukiko, tells of her relationship with the man who was her literature teacher at school, and who is now in his seventies. They meet fortuitously in a tavern and discover that they share similar gastronomic tastes and a fondness for drinking. They continue to see each other at the tavern from time to time by chance. Lonely, heavy drinkers, frugal in conversation and sensitive in nature, they are separated by age and by their interest in culture (his is great, hers is zero).

In the novel, apparently, "nothing happens", there are no great ups and downs, nothing exceptional occurs: only a deep, strong, noticeable relationship is woven, where there is no possibility of anything happening. But what is described is very intense. The teacher no longer expects anything: he has his haikus, the memory of his wife's betrayal, who left him, his peaceful habits. Tsukiko accepts herself as she is, somewhat strange, lonely and restrained.

Kawakami talks about food, drink, walks, short conversations and humour. She gives us only a glimpse into how complicity, admiration, mutual dependence, fondness and love are created. Where do feelings grow from? Where are emotions born? How do these characters, so lonely and defeated, succumb to love?

d. EVERYDAY REFLECTIONS

To read Kawakami is to be carried away by the current of a river on shallow ground. Some things happen because we give them time to do so. Without fright or fanfare.

Some of our projects seem impossible, they are ideas that seem crazy and far from reality. But, if we give them time, if we let the ideas mature, the pieces end up fitting together. The mechanisms are put into motion and the new reality becomes visible.

Ángeles Caso said of Kawakami: "I understand it: her novel is one of the most beautiful love stories I ever have read. I am not referring to one of her books, but to something much deeper and more real, the slow and solid relationship between two lonely beings, in need of each other, capable of finding tenderness and sharing it with their loved one in the midst of the smallest everyday gestures, eating, drinking, going for a walk, sitting by a window in the dark... She narrates in such a delicate and just way that it resembles a piece of real life – maybe it is – painted onto canvas and offered before our eyes to help us become wiser. Read it and enjoy it."

I would say that she is an author for people who understand how to enjoy reading poetry.

e. OTHER RELEVANT FRAGMENTS

"I kept walking towards the station. It was my usual route, but it seemed completely different to me. I had gone back to my childhood. I was like a girl entertaining herself on the way home until it begins to get dark, and when she decides to go back the streets don't seem the same.

'Teacher,' I murmured. 'Teacher, I don't know how to get home.'

But the teacher was not there. As I wondered where he would be that night, I realised that we had never spoken on the phone. We met by chance, we walked together by chance and drank sake by chance. [...] But even if we did not coincide, the teacher was never far from me. He would never be a stranger, and she was sure he was somewhere tonight. Loneliness took hold of me at times, so I decided to sing."

f. SUGGESTED READING

Strange Weather in Tokyo, London, Granta Books, 2013.
The Nakano Thrift Shop, London, Granta Books, 2016.
Yoru no koen (Fragile Lives, Dark Nights), unavailable in English.

The sharp-edged word
of bright pessimism
François de La
Rochefoucauld

a. WHO IS FRANÇOIS DE LA ROCHEFOUCAULD?

François VI, Duc de La Rochefoucauld (Paris, 1613-1680), French aristocrat and military man, was also a writer, known above all for his *Maxims*.

The first part of his life – at the age of sixteen he dropped out of school and enlisted in the army – faithful to a violent nobility who valued war and seduction, was so full of action that he always lived on the frontier of two worlds: death and gambling. Of most noble blood, he could not escape being part of plots against Richelieu or Mazarin. He had a prominent role in the Fronde rebellion, and the war caused him, among other misfortunes, almost complete loss of sight after an injury, and the death of two of his children. After recovering from his wounds, weak, with his fortune diminished and in conflict with the powerful men of his time, he remained in retirement for some years and regained health, fortune and influence, at which time he dedicated himself to leading a totally mundane existence, assiduously frequenting the literary salons.

La Rochefoucauld spent his years of retirement writing his *Maxims* and his *Memoirs* and is considered by many to be the most important of the French moralists.

Context: France in the 17th century was a country of intense risk, war, intrigue, love affairs and the resulting ascents and falls: fortunes inherited and later in some cases, lost. Passion and war, and the discovery of the seduction of noble ladies. Seduction, intrigue and war without end.

La Rochefoucauld had great and powerful enemies, coming from a lineage committed to power, to attaining it and maintaining it, or losing it and trying to regain it.

b. FRAGMENTS OF HIS WORK

"We promise according to our hopes and perform according to our fears."

"The evil that we do does not attract to us so much persecution and hatred as our good qualities."

"Our way of being places value on everything that we owe to luck."

"We are never so happy or unhappy as we think."

"When our hatred is too intense, it puts us on a lower level than those we hate."

"One may outwit another, but not all the others."

c. BRIEF COMMENTARY

To read the **Maxims** of François de La Rochefoucauld is to take a walk through his repertoire of disappointments. Their validity today emanates from the enormous clarity of him contemplating the human condition. His phrases could be a *vade mecum* of cynical thoughts that reality does not appear to easily disprove.

Nietzsche said that he preferred the **Maxims** to "all the books by all the German philosophers."

Large and corrosive, almost nothing remains standing after reading it. He does not idealise himself; he does not idealise others. He knows about love and war, and luck and death. He played hard and with intensity.

d. EVERYDAY REFLECTIONS

In these fierce times we are living, reading François de La Rochefoucauld is like taking your exam to pass the driving test of life. On the side that is, at least: the hardest, the least beautiful, the least idealised, the least clean, the one that leaves us with the bad taste in the mouth of the born survivor.

Reading it is an examination of our innocence. It makes it easier to know how to take sides, because he, although never showing it, allows you, at least, to understand the boundaries between right and wrong with increasing clarity. Reading it is putting yourself to the test.

e. OTHER RELEVANT FRAGMENTS

"Too great haste to repay an obligation is a kind of ingratitude."

"Gratitude is like the good faith of traders: it maintains commerce, and we often pay, not because it is just to discharge our debts, but that we may more readily find people to trust us."

"No one deserves to be praised for kindness if he does not have the strength to be bad; every other form of kindness is most often merely laziness or lack of willpower."

"We often forgive those who have hurt us, but we cannot forgive those who we have hurt us."

"Weak people cannot be sincere."

"Those only are despicable who fear to be despised."

"It is widely known that you do not have to talk much about your own wife, but it is not always taken into account that you should talk even less about yourself."

f. SUGGESTED READING

Mémoires (Memoirs), unavailable in English.
Maxims, London, Penguin Classics, 1982.

Of rural life, simple and authentic, to the most elevated and sublime

Selma Lagerlöf

a. WHO IS SELMA LAGERLÖF?

She was born in 1858 in her family's ancestral home, which was one of the oldest in the Värmland region of Sweden. Much of what she explains about this region has its origin in the legends and stories she was told during her childhood.

Her father went bankrupt and her brother then failed to make the family farm profitable, which had to be given up to pay off debts. Seeing how events were unfolding, Selma decided to prepare herself to earn a living and, thanks to a loan her brother obtained for her, she could study and become a governess. In 1894 he met Sophie Elkan, also a writer, whom she fell deeply in love with and who had a great influence on her.

Her poems, short stories and novels earned her the Nobel Prize for Literature in 1909 – the first time it was awarded to a woman – and shortly after in 1914, she became part of the Swedish Academy.

She eventually managed to recover the ancestral home for her family, where she died in 1940.

Context: A teacher in a small town, and friend to women who were interested in social and feminist issues, Selma Lagerlöf became aware of poverty, alcoholism, dependency, discrimination against women, and their ignorance, and she wrote about it all. A committed feminist, she dedicated much of the 1920s to fighting for women's rights.

The Nazi persecution of German intellectuals was horrific, and Selma Lagerlöf helped writers and thinkers, like author Nelly Sachs, to hide or flee from Germany, and to fight the Nazi dictatorship. In support of the Finnish people, she also became involved in their fight against the Soviet invasion, to the point of auctioning off the Nobel Prize gold medal to raise funds for them. Her efforts to help Finnish refugees sapped her strength and resulted in a massive heart attack, and she died at the home of her birth.

b. FRAGMENTS OF HER WORK

"And there stood Jan, holding in his two hands something soft and warm done up in a big shawl, a corner of which had been turned back that he might see the little wrinkled face and the tiny wizened hands. He was wondering what the womenfolk expected him to do with that which had been thrust upon him, when he felt a sudden shock that shook both him and the child."

"Immediately after, the heart of him began to beat in his breast as it had never done before.

'Say Jan, have you never cared so much for somebody that your heart has been set a throbbing because of her?" asked the midwife.

'No indeed!' said Jan.

But at that moment he knew what it was that had quickened the heart in him. Moreover he was beginning to perceive what had been amiss with him all his life, and that he whose heart does not respond to either joy or sorrow can hardly be called human."

c. BRIEF COMMENTARY

I had been wanting to publish something by Selma Lagerlöf in my company for a long time. Then, in 2018, when, due to scandals, the Nobel Prize for Literature was not awarded, it seemed to me to be the ideal time. She was the first woman to receive this award, and I liked the idea of filling the void left by the Nobel committee with the publication of one of her books that had been least read in Spanish, and which, nevertheless, is a gem that I came to the last page of with tears in my eyes: *The Emperor of Portugalia*.

I'm not going to give away any spoilers, I only wish to explain that the protagonist is a poor man to whom nothing good has ever happened until the day that, when he is older, he has his first daughter – called Klara Fina – and this changes him forever. A luminous transformation takes place.

I think I remember Roland Barthes saying that in all photography there is a place that is the centre, the *punctum*. In ***The Emperor of Portugalia***, the *punctum* is the moment when the old man takes the newborn baby in his arms and for the first time in his life is truly moved by someone. The sensation is so new, that he does not quite understand what is happening to him, he feels his heart beating and for a moment he thinks he is ill, but what is actually taking place is the transforming power of love.

This moment for me is the metaphor, the perfect symbol of what it means to be a father. The moment when you hold a newborn baby in your arms is the moment of maximum maternal feeling that a man can aspire to, and in this novel we are discussing, written by a woman, Jan, the protagonist, is handed this maximum moment of his life, in which his entire existence is given over to love.

There are undercurrents of the great themes of life circulating in this book: the harshness of the countryside, the great cycles of nature, the feeling of justice and the angst of injustice, the poverty, dignity, silence, fear…

A father's love cannot save the poor peasant Jan from worry or financial problems. His daughter is dragged into these circumstances and goes to the city to earn a living to help her parents in a way that will later be perceived as disturbing and ultimately terrible. The book's greatness lies in seeing how Jan cannot stop thinking about her and, in the absence of news, imagines his daughter enjoying a glorious life. His blind trust in Klara's qualities and his obsessive thinking lead him to picture her in a perfect world, of riches, recognition and honours.

Despite the great literary quality of this book, and the other works by Selma Lagerlöf, undoubtedly the most well-known is ***The Wonderful Adventures of Nils***, a work commissioned by the Ministry of Education to teach the geography of her country to children.

It tells the story of Nils, a selfish and spoilt boy who has a spell cast upon him by fairy, who turns him into a child measuring just inches in height. On the back of a goose, he joins a flock of geese on their annual migration north. Nils visits Lapland and travels the length and breadth of Sweden. During the trip, Nils recognises the mistakes he has made and learns to be supportive and not lazy.

As well as having a strong moral tone, the novel teaches a love for nature, geography, culture, mythology and the traditions of the Scandinavian country. The final effect is so successful that when Japanese writer Kenzaburō Oe travelled to Stockholm to collect his Nobel Prize, he spent his free time travelling the country. He stated that as a child, he had read Lagerlöf's work many times, and that everything was just as the author had described in the book.

Another great admirer of the book was Karl Popper, who claimed to have read it at least once a year throughout his life. Konrad Lorenz was also greatly influenced by the adventures of Nils Holgersson. Great books have great readers, who are devoted to these everlasting works.

d. EVERYDAY REFLECTIONS

Lagerlöf speaks to us of the love she has for her country and for simple people. She brings their problems and the bleak reality of their existence to life. She allows you to experience the harsh daily lives of the poorest inhabitants of the countryside.

She honestly and courageously denounces all the injustices she sees, and, through describing them, she makes us want to fight to change them.

A Jesuit priest used to say that one must be on the side of the poor; although they may be in the wrong, those who support them will never be wrong. Lagerlöf stands beside poor people with maximum empathy, as only an honest woman could do: determined, whole, strong, but also empathetic, sensitive and generous.

In reading her work, I think we have a lot to learn from her.

e. OTHER RELEVANT FRAGMENTS

"When Jan of Ruffluck walked home from church the Sunday he had appeared there for the first time in his royal regalia, he turned in on the old forest road. It was a warm sunny day and, as he went up the hill, he heard the music of the spruces so plainly that it astonished him. Never had spruce trees sung like that! It struck him that he ought to find out why they were so loud-voiced just today. And being in no special haste to reach home, he dropped down in the middle of the smooth gravel road, in the shade of the singing tree. Laying his stick on the ground, he removed his cap and mopped his brow, then he sat motionless, with hands clasped, and listened. [...] The instant his head touched the ground and his eyes closed, the trees struck up something new. Ah, now there came rhythm and melody! [...] And now they sang of him— there was no mistaking it now, when they thought him asleep. [...] Ah, this was music! It was not just the young trees at the edge of the road that made music now, but the whole forest. [...] Never had he heard anything so beautiful, nor listened

to music in just this way. It rang in his ear; so that he could never forget it. Immediately he began to sing this hymn of the woods so as to fix it forever in his memory.
The Empress's father, for his part,
Feels so happy in his heart.

f. SUGGESTED READING

The Emperor of Portugalia, Canton, Pinnacle Press, 2017.
The Wonderful Adventures of Nils Holgersson, London, Penguin Classics, 2018.

We read so that we know we are not alone
C. S. Lewis

a. WHO IS C. S. LEWIS?

Clive Staples Lewis was born in Belfast in 1898 and died in Oxford in 1963. He was a professor at the universities of Oxford and Cambridge, a medievalist, renowned literary critic, apologist for Christianity and famous lecturer. He wrote several books of poems, fantasy novels (including the well-known series *The Chronicles of Narnia*), children's stories, essays, and an autobiography. In his memoir, ***Surprised by Joy***, Lewis recalls that he was baptised into the Church of Ireland when he was born, but during his teens he turned his back on his faith. Due to the influence of Tolkien and other friends, Lewis reverted to Christianity in his late thirties, a fact that permeates his work.

In 1956 he married the American writer Joy Gresham, seventeen years his junior, who died of cancer four years later at the age of forty-five. His short book, ***A Grief Observed***, written in 1961 after his wife's death, is a moving read. The memorable film version of this work, ***Shadowlands***, is a masterful recreation of the book and its world. Lewis' works have been translated into more than thirty languages and millions of copies have been sold over the years.

Context: He was born in Belfast, within the Catholic tradition. He became a prominent professor at Oxford, after fighting in the trenches during the First World War, and, after struggling with his own agnosticism, he finally rediscovered his faith.

Erudition and faith form a distinguished spiritual path for C. S. Lewis. Both of these fall apart with the arrival of love and the subsequent traumatic scenario: the death of his beloved wife. No one is prepared for interrupted love. We all celebrate the incursion of love, but we are not prepared for its loss; that is why reading *A Grief Observed* affects how you cherish your loved ones.

b. FRAGMENTS OF HIS WORK

> *"Why is He so present a commander in our time of prosperity and so very absent a help in time of trouble?"*

c. BRIEF COMMENTARY

How is the rational compatible with the spiritual? What good is knowledge when you are suffering? How can you fight with God, when it is He who has helped you before? How can you write about pain, about loss? How can you accompany someone during their greatest defeat?

Reading *A Grief Observed* is to accompany someone in mourning. It is being in the same place and time as the person who is grieving. It is empathising with those who are falling apart and, at the same time, admiring their greatness, their vision, their confrontation with God.

d. EVERYDAY REFLECTIONS

Have you ever had to offer words of condolence and have not known what to say?

Does observing someone else's pain help us to learn something? Do we know how to live when another, whom we love, dies? Do we know how to comfort a person when they have lost someone essential to them? How do we care for them and learn how to comfort them? With words? How do we express our comforting presence with dignity?

A Grief Observed is an incomparable lesson in love, because we see how a believer faces his sorrow, contemplates it and tries to draw conclusions, learn, in his permanent dialogue with himself, with his beloved wife and with God.

When we lose someone essential in our lives, we all look for answers, each in our own way. Even in the reproach of the divine there is an inalienable search for human dignity. As a Jesuit said, in the search for God, it is where He is, even if He is not found.

e. OTHER RELEVANT FRAGMENTS

"Nor have I anything to offer my readers except my conviction that when pain is to be borne, a little courage helps more than much knowledge, a little human sympathy more than much courage, and the least tincture of the love of God more than

all. I write, of course, as a layman of the Church of England: but I have tried to assume nothing that is not professed by all baptised and communicating Christians."

*(In the film **Shadowlands**, there is a memorable moment when he is giving lectures on pain and suffering to Christian teachers and he says:*
"Suffering is the chisel of God to perfect mankind and suffering is that which launches us into the world of others.")

f. SUGGESTED READING

The Chronicles of Narnia, seven volumes, New York, HarperCollins, 2010.
Surprised by Joy, New York, HarperOne, 2017.
The Problem of Pain, New York, HarperCollins, 2001.
A Grief Observed, New York, HarperCollins, 2001.

Two volcanoes of passion in mourning

Rosa Montero

a. WHO IS ROSA MONTERO?

Born in Madrid in 1951, she is a journalist and a key author and icon for many readers.

As a youngster she enjoyed performing with independent theatre groups, such as Canon and Tábano. As a journalist, she collaborated in many media publications (*Fotogramas, Pueblo, Hermano Lobo*…), and since 1977 she has worked for *El País*, although she regularly publishes articles in Latin American and European newspapers.

She stands out as an interviewer and has worked with figures such as Arafat, Palme, Indira Gandhi, Nixon, Cortázar and Malala Yousafzai.

Her work as a professor at various universities, as a scriptwriter for television series or as a presenter have not prevented her from writing nearly fifteen novels, for which she has received many prizes and awards.

She has an honorary doctorate from the University of Puerto Rico and was awarded the National Prize for Spanish Literature, among other outstanding awards.

Context: Rosa, like almost all Spaniards, had to live through the Spanish Transition, a very interesting moment in history in which social, political, economic and technological changes were introduced at great speed. It took people like her, intelligent, lucid, generous and brave, to describe everything that was happening and offer an accurate vision of the steps that men and women were taking to discover their place in a time and country that was bubbling with energy and which was being rebuilt with great talent, will and luck.

b. FRAGMENTS OF HER WORK

"Art in general, and literature in particular, are powerful weapons against Evil and Pain. Novels do not defeat them (they are invincible), but they provide solace for our terror. In the first place, because they unite us with the other humans: literature makes us part of the whole and, in the whole, individual pain seems to hurt a little less. But the spell also works because when suffering breaks our backs, art succeeds in turning that ugly, dirty damage into something beautiful. I narrate and share an excruciating night and in doing so I force sparks of light from the blackness (at least it works for me). That's why Conrad wrote Heart of Darkness: to exorcise and neutralise his experience in the Congo, which was so gruesome it almost drove him mad. That is why Dickens created Oliver Twist and David Copperfield – so that he could endure the suffering of his own childhood. We must do something with all of it, so it does not destroy us, with that roar of despair, with the endless waste, with the furious pain of living when life is cruel. We humans defend ourselves from

senseless pain by adorning it with the wisdom of beauty. We smash coals with our bare hands and sometimes make them look like diamonds."

"'Grief is pure and sacred,' said a nonagenarian to the writer Paul Theroux, and it is a phrase that has been written into my memory. Yes, grief is pure and sacred, and even in death there can be beauty, if we know how to live it."

"Women suffer from the cursed syndrome of redemption.

I think men, on the other hand, tend to be healthier in this respect; they are capable of loving us for who we really are. They don't make up so many things about us, probably because they don't have that much need (for centuries, love has been the only passion that women have been allowed, while men could be passionate about many other things), or maybe they don't have as much imagination. They simply look at us and see us, while we look at them and, in the midst of those first feelings of love, what we see is a delightful fantasy. There is a great phrase from a French comedian named Arthur that reads, "The problem with couples is that women marry thinking that their husbands will change, and men marry thinking that their wives will not."

c. BRIEF COMMENTARY

I have never read an author who is able to combine the macro with the micro quite so well: the world – as big as it is – with the deepest of intimate reflections.

Her life and work reflect a generous devotion to the cause of understanding the feelings of men and women. In *La ridícula idea de no volver a verte* ('The ridiculous idea of never seeing you again'), she offers herself with elegance and rawness, to comment on the life of Madame Curie, and the lives of other women of her time. The life of the two-time Nobel laureate is masterfully interwoven with Rosa's own experiences, some happy, others painful, in a story which is neither trite not overly sentimental. Madame Curie's grief over the death of her husband allows Rosa to portray her own, in a discreet manner, with a good dose of realism and truth. There is an amazing elegance in her writing; a sincerity and intelligence that anything can be spoken of without any sense of shame.

I deeply admire this book by Rosa Montero. Furthermore, it appears in the life of the person who is writing this, always in discreet, intimate, sincere and happy moments. Here I will offer just two examples:

One day I was speaking to Luis Galera, the doctor who brought my three children into the world, about something or other, and when I asked for his opinion, he said to me: "I think what Rosa Montero thinks, as always."

And in this book of Madame Curie, Sarah Dry's important work on the scientist is cited, and Sarah happens to be the daughter of my great friend in America, Paul Dry.

I have great admiration for Rosa Montero. She invites us to learn about the magnificence of other people. With Rosa Montero, no one becomes silent. The words she narrates shine through on their own. When Rosa Montero sets the table, she makes us feel like we are next to her, at home. It is a natural elegance. It is stark nakedness, she does not shy away from showing pain, her writing is lively, intimate, elegant, harsh and comforting all at the same time.

d. EVERYDAY REFLECTIONS

With Rosa Montero we open our eyes and perceive reality with a passion for knowledge. As a good journalist, she investigates and digs deep for information. She analyses it with good judgement and gives praise or criticism honestly, and without fear.

Thanks to her books we remember how to swim, and we immerse ourselves in life, trying to make sense of what surrounds us. It is almost always with humour and affection, but it is also in a serious and rigorous way.

In addition to the doors leading to the outside, there are doors which lead to the inside: what can we say about our emotions, our feelings, of fear, joy, grief or pain?

Lola Beccaria said of her, "While one is reading Rosa Montero's latest book, and then finishes it, the general feeling is one of familiarity and camaraderie. It makes you want to go up to her like an old friend and say: 'Girl, what incredible stories you've been telling me!' And then tie her up so she doesn't escape; force her to continue her story telling, because she has inoculated us with the virus of an unleashed curiosity."

e. OTHER RELEVANT FRAGMENTS

"Real pain is unspeakable. If you can talk about what's causing you pain, you're in luck: it means it's not that important. Because when pain hits you without anything to soften the blow, the first things to be ripped from you are your words."

"Art is a wound turned into light,' said Georges Braque. We need that light, not only those of us who write or paint or compose music, but also those of us who read and see paintings and listen to a concert. We all need beauty to make life bearable. Fernando Pessoa expressed it very well, 'Literature, like art in general, is proof that life is not enough'."

"That is why I also miss knowing the past, the life of Pablo that I did not live. I want to know everything about him. If I could know everything, absolutely everything, it would be as if he had not passed away. We carry our dead on our backs: this is what Amos Oz told me in an interview (Jews have so many dead, he maintained, that the weight is superhuman). Or rather, we are reliquaries of the people we love. We carry them inside us, we are their memory. And we don't want to forget."

f. SUGGESTED READING

La ridícula idea de no volver a verte (The ridiculous idea of not seeing you again), unavailable in English.
El amor de mi vida (The love of my life), unavailable in English.
La loca de la casa (The crazy one of the house), unavailable in English.

There are no obstacles to intelligence

Chimamanda Ngozi Adichie

a. WHO IS CHIMAMANDA NGOZI ADICHIE?

Chimamanda Ngozi Adichie was born in Enugu, Nigeria, in 1977, the fifth daughter of her parents, Grace Ifeoma and James Nwoye. Chimamanda and Ngozi are her first names (meaning 'my God will not fall' and 'blessing', respectively) and Adichie is her surname.

The Adichie family soon moved to Nsukka, home to the University of Nigeria, and lived on the university campus, where her mother was the first woman to be in charge of the admissions department and her father was a professor of statistics. At the age of nineteen, after studying Medicine and Pharmacy for a year and a half in Nsukka, she moved to the United States to study Communication and Political Science at Drexel University (Philadelphia) for two years, after being awarded a scholarship. She then moved to Connecticut, where her sister lived, and in 2001 she graduated with the highest grade: *summa cum laude*.

She also studied creative writing at Johns Hopkins University and received a master's degree in African studies from Yale. Her work as a teacher and her awards and recognitions from the most prestigious North American universities are numerous.

She currently shares her time between Nigeria and the United States, living half the year in each country. She is married and has a daughter.

Her novels, which often feature the cities and surroundings where Chimamanda Ngozi has lived, have received numerous awards and have been translated into more than thirty languages.

Context: Nigeria had gained independence from the British Empire relatively recently, in 1960, when a cruel civil war broke out between 1967 and 1970, as a result of the attempt, in the region where Adichie was born, to gain independence from Nigeria in the name of Biafra.

More than thirty thousand Ibos – the majority ethnic group in Biafra – were massacred and the humanitarian tragedy reached such levels that some doctors who had come to help ended up establishing the NGO *Médecins Sans Frontières*. Chimamanda's family suffered painful losses on both her mother's and her father's side.

During Chimamanda's childhood and youth, Nigeria suffered numerous political upheavals, coups and strikes.

b. FRAGMENTS OF HER WORK

"In Lagos, the harmattan was a mere veil of haze, but in Nsukka it was a raging, mercurial presence; the mornings were crisp, the afternoons ashen with heat, and the nights unknown.

Dust whirls would start in the far distance, very pretty to look at as long as they were far away, and swirl until they coated everything brown. Even eyelashes […]. Some nights, the heat lay like a thick towel. Other nights, sharp cold wind would descend, and Ifemelu would abandon her hostel room and, snuggled next to Obinze on his mattress, listen to the whistling pines howling outside, in a world suddenly fragile and breakable."

"It irked Ifemelu that Bartholomew was not interested in the son of the woman he was courting, and did not bother to pretend that he was. He was jarringly unsuited for, and unworth of, Auntie Uju. A more intelligent man would have realised this and tempered himself, but not Bartholomew. He behaved grandiosely, like a special prize that Auntie Uju was fortunate to have, and she humoured him. Before he tasted the gizzards, he said,

'Let me see if this is any good.'

Auntie Uju laughed and in her laughter was a certain assent, because his words, 'Let me see if this is any good' were about her being a good cook, and therefore a good wife."

"'Why do you have to do this? Your hair was gorgeous braided […].'

'My cool and full hair would work if I were interviewing to be a backing singer in a jazz band, but I need to look professional for this interview, and professional means straight is best […].'

'It's so fucking wrong that you have to do this.'

At night, she struggled to find a comfortable position on her pillow. Two days later, there were scabs on her scalp. Three *days later, they oozed pus. Curt wanted her to see a doctor and she laughed at him. It would heal, she told him, and it did. Later, after she breezed through the job interview, and the woman shook her hand and said she would be 'wonderful fit' in the company, she wondered if the woman would have felt the same way had she walked into that office wearing her thick, kinky, God-given halo of hair, the Afro."*

"Obinze watched him leave. He was going to tick on a form that his client was willing to be removed. "Removed." That word made Obinze feel inanimate. A thing to be removed. A thing without breath and mind. A thing."

c. BRIEF COMMENTARY

I learned of Adichie's existence thanks to her famous TED Talk, where, with her warm, slow voice, and a charismatic presence that revealed her prodigious intelligence, she spoke of the danger of a single narrative: how, when telling just one version about a fact, country or person, we are limiting its complexity and falsifying its reality, which we condemn to oblivion in favour of a poor stereotype.

That is her powerful greatness: Adichie can approach this subject with full knowledge after experiencing it first hand when she came to the United States from her native Nigeria to pursue her university studies.

She is African and her fellow students were convinced that she had lived all her life in a hut, with no running water. They did not understand how she could speak English so well – the official language in Nigeria – or how it could be that one of her favourite singers was Mariah Carey. But as well as that, she was also black! "I did not discover that I was a black girl until I arrived in America," confesses the writer. "In the United States, blackness and success are an oxymoron."

Adichie, who felt secure and confident, beautiful and smart, had to learn how to regain her self-esteem and confidence. Not only that, as a woman she also suffered from incessant gender discrimination.

She has given other TED Talks, such as a very important speech on feminism which has become famous around the world and was made into a very successful little book.

"A feminist is a man or a woman who believes that there should be no discrimination based on gender," she says. She managed to get her slogan, "We should all be feminists", printed onto Dior T-shirts, and Beyoncé has used her words in some of her songs.

Adichie is a born narrator and has a splendid gift for storytelling. In a way which is sewn into reality. Free from theories. She prefers to explain difficult, awkward things in a gentle yet decisive way, using examples from everyday life. As the Elvira Lindo says of her, "She cannot hide her overwhelming talent."

What she achieves is making everything that is discussed seem obvious; she manages to provide reasons with comments that seem innocuous. And if her books of essays are explained and constructed as if they were fiction, her novels allow the reader to become engrossed in her characters and their circumstances – which are new and unusual for the Western reader – and which, at the same time, are harsh and powerful spokespersons of her commitment to the social causes of justice and equality of class, gender and race.

Reading Adichie is verifying that intelligence is the best companion in life and that one can identify injustices, judge them and react to them firmly and without violence, argue without disparagement, and persuade with determination. And that the best weapons that this author possesses are clarity of spirit, irony and generosity.

d. EVERYDAY REFLECTIONS

I now believe that there are people who are born with a special gift for justice and ethics. Why is it that there are those, who from childhood know how to identify what doesn't add up and what is unacceptable? Adichie is like that. She does not torture herself with big questions, she does not over analyse doubts to the point of boredom. She is sharp and cutting, she leaves you unable to reply and, before you know it, you are wearing a T-shirt with her slogan and you would follow her to the end of the world.

She lays bare unequal treatment for reasons of race, sex or nationality, in such a way that it inclines us to spring into action, sets us ethical minimum standards that no one, ever, under any circumstances should question, much less discard. She is a powerful and admirable author. Any WASP (White Anglo-Saxon Protestant) who thinks they are better than she is, is an utter fool.

e. OTHER RELEVANT FRAGMENTS

(From an interview with Claudio Salazar in El País, October 2017)

"My way of being in the world is to tell stories. I am a storyteller. I am interested in the texture of life, not the theories, because theory deflates people, it makes them flat. That's why I don't read about gender theory, I read stories about people."

"The essence of feminism is universal and at the same time very specific. Many of those books speak of experiences that I cannot relate to. My feminism was born because, even as a child, I remember being told that I could not participate in certain rituals, typical of my culture, because I was a woman. I remember thinking that it didn't make sense. I grew up surrounded by brave women and I noticed that we are always acting. I have seen some very strong women who change in the presence of men. I was always aware of it so obviously there is a part of me who is interested in women's stories."

f. SUGGESTED READING

Americanah, New York, HarperCollins, 2014.
Half of a Yellow Sun, New York, HarperCollins, 2003.
We Should All Be Feminists, New York, HarperCollins, 2014.

A harsh and corrosive vision of the world of work in Japan
Amélie Nothomb

a. WHO IS AMÉLIE NOTHOMB?

Amélie Nothomb is the pseudonym of Fabienne Claire Nothomb, a Belgian writer born in 1966, endowed with a special character and temperament, due in part to various circumstances in her life.

Firstly, she came from a noble family and some of her ancestors were prominent people in the political and cultural spheres of her country, Belgium.

Likewise, she was influenced by the constant changes in her living environment, as her father was a diplomat and travelled with her family to various destinations to live: Osaka, Beijing, New York, Laos, Bangladesh and Burma.

Amélie therefore grew up in exotic and special environments. In fact, she did not return to Belgium until she was seventeen years old, and there she needed some time to integrate, partly because she came from a family with political weight, who were Catholic and right-wing, in part due to the many years they had lived in the East.

She graduated in Philology and returned to Japan, where, at the time, her father was an ambassador. There she worked as an intern, as an interpreter in a Japanese company, which inspired her to write two novels. One of which, **Fear and Trembling**, we will look at in more detail.

Since 1992, Amélie Nothomb has published one book a year, even though she says she writes many more, up to three or four a year. Her stories are lively, and through her rich and creative language she was elected as a member of the Academy of French language and literature of Belgium. The themes she chooses are extremely original and surprising, but perhaps what most characterises and defines her is her sharpness, how caustic she can be, and at times relentless, cold and ironic. At the same time, she is capable of creating absurd worlds, full of poetry, with her very subtle humour, which is almost always provocative. Her originality is the result of her eccentric life straddling East and West, her audacity, her unquestionable deep-rooted intelligence, the generations of culture, of long journeys and unusual experiences.

Context: Amélie Nothomb lives in Brussels, although she often travels to Paris, where she has been given her own office in Albin Michel publishing house. She has links to associations which support women's equality and continues to monitor the rise of the extreme right, also in France.

She also remains connected to her beloved Japan. It is worth noting the generosity that the author showed by donating all her rights to the special edition of **Fear and Trembling** to the victims of the 2011 earthquake and tsunami in Japan.

b. FRAGMENTS OF HER WORK

"Mister Saito summoned me to his office. I was treated to a well-deserved telling-off. I had committed the crime of showing initiative. I had taken a function upon myself without asking for permission from my direct superiors."

"To think that I had been silly enough to get a college degree. There can be nothing less intellectually stimulating than repetition. I was devoted to order, not thought, I now realized. Writing down numbers while contemplating beauty was happiness itself. […] My mind was not that of a conqueror, but that of a cow that spends its life chewing contentedly in the meadow of invoices, waiting for the train of eternal grace to pass by. How good it felt to exist without pride or ambition. To live in hibernation."

"Not all Japanese women are beautiful. But when one of them sets out to be beautiful, anyone else had better stand back.

All forms of beauty are poignant, Japanese beauty particularly so. That lily-white complexion, those mellow eyes, the inimitable shape of the nose, the well-defined contours of the mouth, and the complicated sweetness of the features are enough, by themselves, to eclipse the most perfectly assembled faces. Finally, and most importantly, beauty that has resisted so many physical and mental corsets, so many constraints, crushing denials, absurd restrictions, dogmas, heartbreaks, such sadism and asphyxiation, and such conspiracies of silence and humiliation—that sort of beauty is a miracle of heroic survival."

"Ah, but there is one! Just one. One to which you [the Japanese woman], have every right to avail yourself—unless you have been stupid enough to convert to Christianity. You have the right to commit suicide. Suicide is a very honourable act. [...] Granted, you can choose not to commit suicide. But then, sooner or later, you will find you can no longer cope, and slip into some form or other of dishonour: take a lover, indulge gluttony, grow lazy. It has been observed that humans in general, and women in particular, find it hard to exist for any length of time without succumbing to one of these carnal pleasures. If we are wary, it will not be out of Puritanism. That is an American obsession. It is best to avoid any kind of physical pleasure, because it is apt to make you sweat. There is nothing more shameful than sweat."

"The content was incredibly insulting. My companion in misfortune and I were called traitors, incompetents, snakes, deceitful, and—the height of injury— individualists. The delivery explained much about Japanese history. I would have been capable of anything to stop the hideous screaming—invade Manchuria, persecute millions of Chinese, commit suicide for the Emperor, hurl my airplane into an American battleship, perhaps even work for two Yumimoto Corporations."

"I was somehow not sufficiently unwise to let myself do what, in other circumstances, would have been a normal reflex: to intervene. There is no doubt it would have aggravated the situation—for both the sacrificial lamb and for me. And yet I cannot pretend I felt proud of myself. Honour sometimes means doing something very unwise. Behaving like an idiot is better than dishonour. To this day I blush for having chosen sensible restraint over common decency. Someone should have

done something; and since there was no chance the others would have put themselves at risk, it should have been me."

c. BRIEF COMMENTARY

The title of her book ***Fear and Trembling*** refers to the attitude one was supposed to have towards the Japanese emperor. Something quite incomprehensible to our Western eyes and, for that matter, wisely disregarded today. In Japan, however, the attitude of extreme humiliation had to be shown physically through trembling!

A great connoisseur of the country and its language, the young Amélie goes to work in a Japanese company and astounds us with a ludicrous account of how traditional Japanese values are embedded in the company. Her quick-witted ability to unravel the envy, abuse of power, humiliation, meaningless work, contradictions and the (terrible) situation of women. The beautiful image of the Shinto garden is all very well, but the world of work, as described by her, leaves you feeling dazed.

She only talks about the world of work. At no time does her story leave the office. Her intention is to endure job for a year. On one hand she surrenders to this idea, and on the other she mentally distances herself from the ludicrous nonsense of which she is sometimes witness and sometimes victim.

It is a vicious and amusing critique of a Japanese company. But we should try to imagine what would happen if one day a Japanese woman came to work in a European company... How would she paint a picture of some of our office customs?

Nothomb states that everything that she writes about in

the book is one hundred percent true. She says, "It's a story for which I needed no imagination. In 1990 I actually worked there, it was one of the biggest Japanese companies at the time." "Yes, this book is a little payback towards Japanese company culture, but it is nothing against Japan at all."

d. EVERYDAY REFLECTIONS

Sometimes stuck in an office, often for too long (prisoners of work presenteeism), we have created an underworld with its own rules. But let's be wary: the dynamics of human passions at times live in parallel to the genuine interests of the business: envy, abuse, offensive comments…

It is incredible how Nothomb, knowing how young she was then, knew perfectly how to capture this underworld with its own rules, and portray the characters that had been trapped within it. And anyone who enters this underworld ends up getting caught up in it: Amélie herself spends three sleepless nights in the office, trying to balance some representation expenses. Three nights in a row! It is one of my favourite scenes, because of how ludicrous and funny it is, because of how over the top and out of control the situation is. You think it's delirium, and then it turns out to be true.

The perversion of the system leads employees to believe that they must sacrifice their time to achieve goals that we find trivial and silly, as well as very unhealthy. (In Japan, according to many media sources, many employees fall ill from poor sleep.)

e. OTHER RELEVANT FRAGMENTS

"I remembered a line from André Maurois: "Don't speak too ill of yourself. People will believe you."

"What awaited these poor number-crunchers outside The Company? The obligatory beer with colleagues undergoing the same kind of gradual lobotomy, hours spent stuffed into an overcrowded subway, a dozing wife, sleep that sucked them down into it like the vortex of a flushing toilet, the occasional day off they never took full advantage of. Nothing that deserved to be called a life. The worst part of it all was that they were considered lucky."

f. SUGGESTED READING

Hygiene and the Assassin, London, Europa Editions, 2010.
The Book of Proper Names, New York, St. Martin's Press, 2004.
Pétronille, London, Europa Editions, 2015.

The value of hope
Octavio Paz

a. WHO IS OCTAVIO PAZ?

Octavio Paz (Mexico, 1914-1998), winner of the Cervantes Prize in 1981 and the Nobel Prize for Literature in 1990, was one of the greatest poets, essayists and translators of the 20th century. His childhood was shaped by the political activity of his father, a notary and Emiliano Zapata's lawyer. He was a writer with a vocation for it from a young age, and his adolescence and youth were marked by his political commitment to his country and to communism, and by his relationship with the culture of Mexico in turmoil. Among other things, he attended the Second International Congress of Antifascist Writers in July 1937, which was held in Valencia. A Guggenheim Fellowship enabled him to study at Berkeley in 1943. He completed his experience abroad with time spent in India and Japan. In 1945 he joined the Mexican diplomatic corps and participated in the surrealist movement in Paris. He was the Mexican ambassador to India between 1962 and 1968 and resigned from his post after the Tlatelolco massacre. He also worked as a professor at universities in the United States. He was the founder of the Taller, Plural and Vuelta magazines. He met some of the greatest exponents of world literature at the time, such as Neruda and Vallejo, before becoming one himself.

Context: Octavio Paz forms part of a group of poets and thinkers marked by a vast culture, a real cosmopolitanism and a unique knowledge of East and West. Educated, committed, brave and wise, he is a poet who was tied to the world's cultural elite. The list of awards and distinctions he received demonstrates the enormous international respect he earned, and his translations form a fundamental part of his work.

b. FRAGMENTS OF HIS WORK

"After chopping off all the arms that reached out to me; after boarding up all the windows and doors; after filling all the pits with poisoned water; after building my house on the rock of no, inaccessible to flattery and fear; after cutting off my tongue and eating it; after hurling handfuls of silence and monosyllable of scorn at my loves; after forgetting my name; and the name of my birthplace; and the name of my race; after judging and sentencing myself to perpetual waiting, and perpetual loneliness, I heard against the stones of my dungeon of syllogisms, the humid, tender, insistent onset of spring."

c. BRIEF COMMENTARY

It is not easy to find the greatest authors, of great culture, who bring hope. Frequently, pessimism, dissent, alcohol, anguish or lucidity seem to encourage us to see everything negatively, except in the case of some thinkers or creators who have been saved by the hand of love, optimism, faith, commitment or goodness.

It often seems that pessimism adds a touch of refinement. And yet, in this fragment of *Eagle or Sun?*, Paz's text is filled with bright light, like a sky bursting with sunshine after heavy a downpour.

Occasionally authors such as Auden and his redemption through love, or Torga and his tender and solitary luminosity, can give us faith to live and survive the most devastating of storms.

Coming across a text like this, either by destiny or by chance, illustrates that life can sometimes give us an unexpected lesson in beauty and energy.

d. EVERYDAY REFLECTIONS

Each one of us can decide what to do, what to think, what to expect, and what to feel. As much as there are times when the cold freezes us or the sun burns us, not even the South Pole or the Atacama Desert can take away the elegance of our attitude: the choice of how we will live, survive, defend ourselves, celebrate or how we will suffer adversity, defeat or victory.

When a thirty-seven-year-old poet publishes a book like *Eagle or Sun?*, he could well say that he has lived a complete life. In Octavio Paz we find an immense number of pages filled with diverse topics that give us the key to understanding why culture is a pleasure when it is given to us and when we know how to accept and enjoy it.

Paz is a challenge because he is a world in himself; therefore, even in a small corner of it we will find complete meaning, as in any great work of art.

e. OTHER RELEVANT FRAGMENTS

«Al prefecto Chang
Mi otoño: entro en la calma,
lejos el mundo y sus peleas.
No más afán que regresar,
desaprender entre los árboles.
El viento del pinar abre mi capa,
mi flauta saluda a la luna serrana.
Preguntas, ¿qué leyes rigen "éxito" y "fracaso"?
Cantos de pescadores flotan en la ensenada.»

WANG WEI, TRANSLATED BY OCTAVIO PAZ*

"He wanted to sing, to sing
to forget
his true life of lies
and to remember
his lying life of truths."

f. SUGGESTED READING

The Bow and the Lyre, Austin, University of Texas Press, 2013.
The Double Flame, Boston, Houghton Mifflin Harcourt, 1995.
The Monkey Grammarian, New York, Arcade Publishing, 2017.
In Light of India, Boston, Mariner Books, 1998.
Eagle or Sun?, Cambridge, New Directions Publishing, 1976.
The Labyrinth of Solitude, London, Penguin Books, 2008

---

* Answering Vice-Prefect Zhang/As the years go by, give me but peace,/Freedom from ten thousand matters./I ask myself and always answer:/What can be better than coming home?/A wind from the pine-trees blows my sash,/And my lute is bright with the mountain moon./You ask me about good and evil fortune?/Hark, on the lake there's a fisherman singing!

An encounter with spirituality
Jacques Philippe

a. WHO IS JACQUES PHILIPPE?

Jacques Philippe was born in 1947 in Lorraine, France. After studying mathematics at university, he spent several years teaching and doing scientific research. In 1976 he met with the newly founded Community of the Beatitudes and answered the call of faith. He spent several years in Nazareth and Jerusalem, immersing himself in the study of Hebrew and the Jewish roots of Christianity. In 1981 he travelled to Rome to study Theology and Canon Law, was ordained a priest in 1985 and began his work as a spiritual director, training priests and seminarians in the community. In 1994 he returned to France, where he assumed various responsibilities, including the development of teaching in the community and participation in its General Council. He has also regularly led retreats in France and abroad, and his main themes have been written as various books on spirituality, of which he has sold more than a million copies in twenty-four languages.

His writings deal with topics such as prayer, inner freedom and peace of the heart. His extraordinary diffusion has made him a classic of modern Catholic spirituality. In recent years he has devoted himself mainly to spiritual direction and leading spiritual retreats.

Context: The religious theme of the book and its author can be placed within a framework of especially interesting origin, France; a country which separated the Church from the State after the revolution. That's quite something. Theocracies today are the source of some of the most disturbing issues of our time.

Interest in its context grows because France is the country where the author was born. As well as this, France is one of the most cultured countries in the world, and the end of World War II means putting Adorno's phrase – that it is impossible to write poetry after Auschwitz – to the test. Poetry and spirituality are often closely linked to each other.

To understand Jacques Philippe and his environment, we can turn to the thoughts of another Frenchman, none other than André Malraux, who was a great writer and the Minister of Culture of France with De Gaulle, who was linked to the following phrase in a speech: "The 21st century will be religious or it will not be."

This is not the phrase word for word, something which Malraux himself would also agree with. However, this variation does belong to him: "The 21st century will be spiritual or it will not be." In any case, two of Malraux's thoughts were also documented, formulated at the end of World War II, shortly before Jacques Philippe was born, which are of interest to us because of the author, subject and book we are dealing with.

"For fifty years psychology has reintegrated demons into man. Such is the serious assessment of psychoanalysis. I think that the task of the next century, in the face of the most terrible threat that humanity has known, will be to reintroduce the gods there."

> *"The central problem of the end of the century will be the religious problem – in a form as different from that which we know, as Christianity was from the ancient religions."*

The bases have been established for both searching and finding (or not).

b. FRAGMENTS OF HIS WORK

> *"We have this great thirst for freedom because our most fundamental aspiration is for happiness; and we sense that there is no happiness without love, and no love without freedom. This is perfectly true. Human beings were created for love, and they can only find happiness in loving and being loved. As St. Catherine of Siena puts it, man cannot live without loving. The problem is that our love often goes in the wrong direction: we love ourselves, selfishly, and end up frustrated, because only genuine love can fulfill us."*

> *"Our lack of freedom comes from our lack of love: we believe we are victims of an unfavourable context when the real problem (and with it, its solution) is found within us."*

> *"Freedom is not only choosing, but accepting what we have not chosen."*

> *"I would like to highlight the importance of this way of exercising freedom. The highest and most fruitful act of human freedom resides in acceptance rather than domination. Man manifests the greatness of his freedom when he transforms reality, but even more so when he confidently accepts the reality that comes to him day after day."*

c. BRIEF COMMENTARY

Jacques Philippe is an immense author. ***Interior Freedom*** is much more than a religious book (as if this were not enough). It is a book of moving luminosity and joy, as the subtitle also reveals: *The strength of faith, hope and love*. I think I used up a third of my pencil underlining such a huge number of pages in this gem of a book.

Every human being has the possibility to wonder (or not) about the spiritual and religious phenomenon. Both options are equally respectable. Some people have faith. Others, even if they don't, may share the desire of those with faith to ask and wonder about transcendence. About what is right. About what is good. About what is true.

The area of faith, even though it brings people together in many cases, includes as many possibilities as there are individual responses for each person. In any case, for many people, an expression of believing can respond to a need, as much as or even more than, a decision. There are as many possibilities as there are believers, and ways for people to experience transcendence.

Faith and beliefs are not types of ideologies, something that is received and to which one simply says "yes", maybe forever. Faith and beliefs are realities that respond to a deep dimension which is inherent in almost every human being: the need for spirituality. It is one that is gaining strength everywhere – even in our non-believing West – even though religion and spirituality do not always go together with the symmetrical precision of an engineer.

There is probably more plurality among believers than among agnostics, although no one would know. Because, like so many essential things in life, they tend to be private. And each individual is alone (or accompanied) in their own way.

Living without faith is possible, though perhaps the experience can be likened to being in the desert without any shade.

Lucidity being desirable to some, and at the same time a lethal mutation to others, does not exempt us from seeking answers, beyond our own life and field of vision.

Albert Camus said that collectives must be judged according to the characteristics of the best people in that group. Well, believers, at their best, are people to look up to. Feeling a great deal of warmth or respect towards them is natural. It is worth being around them. Reach out to them and investigate.

d. EVERYDAY REFLECTIONS

It is helpful to reserve a quiet space for the following thought: the most profound thing we can do today, to seek out the best in ourselves, is perhaps none of the following, very reasonable, options: do yoga, practise mindfulness, learn how to eat better, drink herbal teas, walk in the mountains, sleep better, perform theatre, sing, take a stroll…

All these options are admirable and, without a doubt, can provide you with a path and the foundations for a more fulfilled life. However, perhaps it can also leave us space and time – whether before or after – totally or partially, to experience transcendency.

Opening ourselves up to an essential topic in human life: religiosity, transcendence – whatever it is and however it is called. Do it, if you feel up to it, if you can, if you decide to, in a very delicate and, I should add, private way. When it happens, if it happens, it is helpful to have a clear mind and an open spirit, opening the door to your own freedom.

e. OTHER RELEVANT FRAGMENTS

"This is the point – of decisive importance – that we are going to address now: to achieve true interior freedom we must train ourselves to accept, peacefully and willingly, plenty of things that seem to contradict our freedom. This means consenting to our personal limitations, our weaknesses, our powerlessness, this or that situation that life imposes on us, and so on. We find it difficult to do this, because we feel a natural revulsion for situations we cannot control. But the fact is that the situations that really make us grow are precisely those we do not control; and we will illustrate it with a good number of particular examples."

"We will advance much more securely and efficiently if we fully deliver ourselves to the good of which we are capable, despite our failures, than by worrying excessively about them."

"Pain is fruitful and can make life beautiful."

f. SUGGESTED READING

Interior Freedom, Strongsville, Scepter Publishers, 2007.
Searching for and Maintaining Peace, New York, Alba House, 2014.

A perfection in nuances
Josep Pla

a. WHO IS JOSEP PLA?

Josep Pla was born in Palafrugell in 1897, and died in Llofriu in 1981, two towns in the province of Girona. He was a prolific Spanish writer and journalist in the Catalan and Spanish languages. He is in fact the most relevant prose author of the 20th century Catalan literature. He graduated in law in 1919 and began working as a journalist. He revealed himself to be an exceptional witness of his time, from many angles and places. He lived in Madrid during the Second Spanish Republic and served as a correspondent for *La Veu* (1931-1936). He travelled all over the world and published numerous articles for *Destino* magazine between 1939 and 1976. Josep Pla gives his name to one of the most important literary awards in the Catalan language.

Context: Pla was a journalist who was alive throughout most important events of the 20th century: he lived in Paris during his personal exile, from Madrid he was a witness to the establishment of the Second Spanish Republic and lived through the post-war period, travelling to the Soviet Union, France, Israel, New York and South America.

To speak of Pla is to see how an intelligent spirit, with an ability to write for the public, lives alongside the turmoil of unfolding events. It is his meticulous passion for detail of the vision he interprets. He comments on the history of the great and the small, demonstrating the accuracy of this phrase by Rainer Maria Rilke (1875-1926).

> *"Because in the same way that big is big,*
> *small is not small."*

b. FRAGMENTS OF HIS WORK

> *"If you get the adjectives right, the writer exists."*

> *"I believe that, in effect, almond trees are a thing of poetry, they are beautiful figurations. They are a thing of such beauty that when, by virtue of the transience of things, the petals fall, I feel the same fundamental emptiness that I felt that day in Cagliari, in Sardinia, my wallet was stolen."*

c. BRIEF COMMENTARY

Pla is a writer of enormous richness and intelligence. He is one of the greatest figures in Catalan literature of the last century. He is brilliant, distant, frank, disconcerting, rich in nuance (this is his essence) and, above all, real.

This attachment to reality is what always makes him lean towards transparent literature, based on "intelligibility, clarity and simplicity."

His observations on the world are always so sharp that one reads Pla with an admiration devoid of envy; the admiration one has for someone who is recognised as a superior writer.

d. EVERYDAY REFLECTIONS

Reading Pla stimulates your outlook on the world. He can create poetry full of reality when he describes how wonderful it is to crush a grape between your teeth and, with it, make the moment beautiful, because he has made you aware of it.

His comments on people, countries, food, thoughts, writers, etc., are as delicious as the first bite of bread. And sometimes they cut like a knife.

To read Pla is to learn how to look at the world.

e. OTHER RELEVANT FRAGMENTS

"What is seny? Ultimately, it consists of separating the difference between the two extremes, which is nothing other than commercial technique."

"Italians are not what they seem. Their coldness is absolute, they sing opera to sell tickets."

"My theory is that happiness is nothing more than receiving a bonus. Something that is given to us randomly."

"Man is a very lonely being, but the only thing that allows him to escape a bit of loneliness is marriage. Especially when there are children."

"To be happy in this world you should not be envious."

"Russia is nothing more than a trend towards the poor becoming rich and the rich becoming poor."

"I believe in travelling by boat. I am an advocate not of progress, but of going back to where you came from. Little by little, all in good time… paying attention to what you're doing, keeping things in mind."

"Revolutions are useless."

"Authors to read: Pascal, La Bruyère, La Rochefoucauld and Montaigne."

"In general, people have too many friends."

"Everything goes up and down, everything will go down."

f. SUGGESTED READING

El carrer estret ('The Narrow Street'), unavailable in English.
The Gray Notebook, New York, NYRB Classics, 2014.

An unrivalled story teller
Katherine Anne Porter

a. WHO IS KATHERINE ANNE PORTER?

Katherine Anne Porter was born in Indian Creek, Texas, in 1890, and died in Maryland in 1980. She was a journalist, writer of novels and short stories, essayist, and winner of the 1966 Pulitzer Prize and National Book Award for *The Collected Stories*. In 1967 she was awarded a gold medal from the American Academy of Arts and Letters. She was also nominated three times for the Nobel Prize in Literature. She lost her mother when she was two years old, grew up in poverty and was barely able to study. She was raised by her paternal grandmother, and shortly after her death, Porter married at the age of sixteen. The marriage, her first of four, was disastrous. She was not able to have children. Between 1920 and 1930 she lived in places such as New York, and also settled in Mexico, where she came into contact with the revolution, of which she became disillusioned.

Her life was marked by a limitless determination, and at the same time by a constant overcoming of adversities; whether it was the burden of her fragile health (she was mistakenly diagnosed with tuberculosis and treated for two years), her unhappy marriages or the price of living with such passion.

All this made her realise the harshness of the world. Her name and popularity lasted two decades, from roughly 1930 to 1950. Her 1962 work, ***Ship of Fools***, was the highest-selling novel in the United States that year and was made into a film by Stanley Kramer in 1965. It tells of a trip from Mexico to Europe which ends in Hitler's Berlin. Her short stories were always well received by critics and her work was highly praised by Truman Capote and Robert Penn Warren.

Separated from the Catholic religion, she returned to it again before her death. Her ashes are buried next to her mother in the Indian Creek Cemetery in Texas.

Context: Porter was born in Texas into poverty, she moved around the United States, she felt a deep understanding and commitment to social issues, she worked as a journalist during World War I, she barely survived the 1918 flu epidemic, she resided in Greenwich Village in New York in its bohemian and radical heyday, she lived in Mexico during a failed revolution, she was there in Europe during the rise of Nazism, and then returned to America during the Cold War and McCarthyism. Taking all this into account, there is little chance that someone like her could produce dull and uninspiring stories. Nothing will be friendly or hospitable.

This iron-willed author made her way from Texas to the world through her words and deeds. She was fearless and overcame the vicissitudes of life with a corrosive prose. A turbulent love life, full of raucous breakups and extremely tough experiences of miscarriage, and even a stillbirth. It was not an easy existence.

She withstood the harshness of life with little comfort to hand. As she herself described, "I've only spent about ten percent of my energies on writing. The other ninety percent went to keeping my head above water."

b. FRAGMENTS OF HER WORK

"In this moment she felt that she had been robbed of an enormous number of valuable things, whether material or intangible: things lost or broken by her own fault, things she had forgotten and left in houses when she moved: books borrowed from her and not returned, journeys she had planned and had not made, words she had waited to hear spoken to her and had not heard, and the words she meant to answer with bitter alternatives and intolerable substitutes worse than nothing, and yet inescapable: the long patient suffering of dying friendships and the dark inexplicable death of love - all that she had, and all that she had missed, were lost together, and were twice lost in this landslide of remembered losses."

c. BRIEF COMMENTARY

Reading novels takes time. Reading short stories on the other hand, requires a generosity from the reader. A desire to delve into the story with curiosity and dedication; to make an incision in time, and into the world. It is brief, intense, full of details hidden between the lines. Be attentive because many things happen within a small space. Someone offers you their life, piece by piece. Sometimes it is a life in pieces. In **War and Peace** an entire world unravels before our eyes, you could live your whole life with its characters. But in a short story, someone throws you a grenade and it explodes, apparently without sound, like in a silent film: the shock wave of a life unfolds when you read a short story. Its rapid spread astounds you.

Katherine Anne Porter's short stories are written with an elegant, yet harsh, prose. They feature a world of characters torn between a thirst for justice, violence, betrayal, disillusionment, sensuality and impossible redemption. Just like the author's life, their reading is not for people used to easy living, whose only map of the world is their living room sofa (both physically and metaphorically).

Katherine Anne Porter will leave you sitting on the floor. Nothing is soft.

d. EVERYDAY REFLECTIONS

A life, which has been really lived, can be expressed in many ways. To offer two (caricatured) extremes, it can be portrayed in a way which is generous and understanding; full of acceptance, like the life of a Tibetan lama who gives you peace, love, understanding and acceptance. It can also be expressed in a way which is more fractured; extreme in its forms, modes and expression – as in an Elizabeth Taylor film – it can resemble a knife.

Theft, by K. A. Porter, is like a blow that knocks you to the ground. It is reminiscent of the phrase by the German author Georg Büchner: "A single drop of pain tears the universe from top to bottom."

It leaves you lying there, alone on the ground. In the company of people you don't know. It has made you older.

Christmas is over. Father Christmas isn't real. They killed Bambi's mother. The big bad wolf doesn't only exist in stories.

e. OTHER RELEVANT FRAGMENTS

"We are more alike than you realize in some things. Wait and see."

"She is not at home in the world. Everyday she teaches children who remain strangers to her, although she loves their tender round hands and their charming opportunistic savagery. She knocks at unfamiliar doors, not knowing whether a friend or a stranger shall answer, and even if a known face emerges from the sour gloom, still is the face of a stranger. No matter what this stranger says to her, nor what her message to him, the very cells of her flesh reject knowledge and kinship in one monotonous word. No. No. No. She draws her strength from this one holy talismanic word which does not suffer her to be led into evil. Denying everything, she may walk anywhere in safety, she looks at everything without amazement."

"[…] the almost ecstatic death-expectancy which is in the air of Mexico. The Mexican may know when the danger is real, or may not care whether the trill is false or true, but strangers feel the acid of death in their bones whether or not any real danger is near them. It was this terror that Kennerly had translated into fear of food, water, and air around him. In the Indian the love of death had become a habit of the spirit. It had smoothed out and polished the faces to a repose so absolute it seemed studied, though studied for so long it was held now without effort; and in them was all a common memory of defeat. The pride of their bodily posture was the mere outward shade of passive, profound

resistance; the lifted arrogant features were a mockery of the servants who lived within."

f. SUGGESTED READING

Flowering Judas, New York, Signet Classics, 1970.
Collected Stories, Boston, Houghton Mifflin Harcourt, 1970.
Ship of Fools, Boston, Little Brown and Company, 1988.

See the essential

Antoine de Saint-Exupéry

a. WHO IS ANTOINE DE SAINT EXUPÉRY?

Antoine de Saint-Exupéry (Lyon, 1900 - some unknown place in the Mediterranean, 1944) was a French writer and aviator. He was born into an aristocratic family and had a happy childhood, although the premature death of his father deeply affected the entire family. He worked as a pilot in the Spanish Sahara and later in Buenos Aires, where he was appointed director of Aeroposta Argentina and was in charge of organising the aviation network in Latin America. In 1931 he married the Salvadoran Consuelo Suncín, with whom he had a complicated relationship, which is said to have inspired his book *The Little Prince*.

When Aeroposta closed, Saint-Exupéry flew as a test pilot and made several record attempts. He suffered two serious accidents: in the Egyptian desert in 1935 and in Guatemala in 1938.

During World War II he fought with the French airforce. After the fall of France he went to New York. As of 1943, he asked to join the French forces in North Africa and resumed missions from Sardinia and Corsica. On July 31, 1944, his plane disappeared in the Mediterranean.

His written work always reflected his passion for flying.

Context: France and the first half of the 20th century. A life marked by his passion for piloting, his love for people and the Second World War. A happy childhood and a country at war. His passion for flying was the leitmotif of his life.

b. FRAGMENTS OF HIS WORK

"It was then that the fox appeared.

'Good morning,' said the fox.

'Good morning,' the little prince responded politely, although when he turned around he saw nothing.

'I am right here,' the voice said, 'under the apple tree.'

'Who are you?' asked the little prince, and added, 'You are very pretty to look at.'

'I am a fox,' the fox said.

'Come and play with me,' proposed the little prince. 'I am so unhappy.'

'I cannot play with you,' the fox said. 'I am not tamed.'

'Ah! Please excuse me,' said the little prince. But, after some thought, he added: 'What does that mean—tame?'

'You do not live here,' said the fox. 'What is it that you are looking for?'

'I am looking for men,' said the little prince. 'What does that mean—tame?'

'Men,' said the fox. 'They have guns, and they hunt. It is very disturbing. They also raise chickens. These are their only interests. Are you looking for chickens?'

'No,' said the little prince. 'I am looking for friends. What does that mean—tame?'

'It is an act too often neglected,' said the fox. It means to establish ties.'

'To establish ties?'

'Just that,' said the fox. 'To me, you are still nothing more than a little boy who is just like a hundred thousand other little boys. And I have no need of you. And you, on your part, have no need of me. To you, I am nothing more than a fox like a hundred thousand other foxes. But if you tame me, then we shall need each other. To me, you will be unique in all the world. To you, I shall be unique in all the world…'"

c. BRIEF COMMENTARY

The Little Prince, one of the world's greatest bestsellers, has sold more than 140 million copies worldwide since 1943 and has been translated into more than 250 languages.

Where lies the greatness of this text, one of the most widely read works of humanity?

It is a true masterpiece of a children's story, but also particularly for adults, since it is an invitation to rethink our way of looking at the world that, far from losing relevance, is more pertinent than ever.

The tenderness, delicacy, rawness and sadness that some of its pages exude have been moving us for more than seventy years, proving that a classic is what remains when neither time nor space can wear it away.

d. EVERYDAY REFLECTIONS

We are moved by the enormous simplicity and depth of its pages, and its reading continues to serve as the ultimate test to know if we are becoming hardened. He who reads it with indifference is someone who has probably given up, who has lost the ability to look at the world with the naked eyes of a child and to ask questions. Reading it without feeling emotion is such a strange concept that perhaps someone who does not feel this emotion cannot identify the essentials of life.

In most cases, reading **The Little Prince** with indifference is possibly a sign that they need to visit a therapist.

e. OTHER RELEVANT FRAGMENTS

"The fox gazed at the little prince, for a long time.
'Please—tame me!' he said.
'I want to, very much,' the little prince replied. 'But I have not much time. I have friends to discover, and a great many things to understand.'
'One only understands the things that one tames,' said the fox. 'Men have no more time to understand anything. They buy things all ready made at the shops. But there is no shop anywhere where one can buy friendship, and so men have no friends any more. If you want a friend, tame me ...'
'What must I do, to tame you?' asked the little prince.
'You must be very patient,' replied the fox. 'First you will sit down at a little distance from me— like that— in the grass. I shall look at you out of the corner of my eye, and you will say nothing. Words are the source of misunderstandings. But you will sit a little closer to me, every day ...'

The next day the little prince came back.

'It would have been better to come back at the same hour,' said the fox. 'if, for example, you come at four o'clock in the afternoon, then at three o'clock I shall begin to be happy. I shall feel happier and happier as the hour advances. At four o'clock, I shall already be worrying and jumping about. I shall show you how happy I am! But if you come at just any time, I shall never know at what hour my heart is to be ready to greet you . . . One must observe the proper rites . . .'"

f. SUGGESTED READING

Wind, Sand and Stars, Boston, Harcourt, 2002.
Night Flight, Boston, Mariner Books, 1974.
The Little Prince, Egmont Books, Glasgow, 2004.

He can break your heart
with a sentence
James Salter

a. WHO IS JAMES SALTER?

James Salter was born in 1925 in New York, he studied engineering at West Point, and in 1945 started in the Air Force. He was a fighter jet pilot and fought in the Korean War. He died in Sag Harbor, New York state, in 2015. In 1956, at the age of thirty-two, he published his first book, *The Hunters*, and a year later he left the Army to devote himself to literature. For a decade he worked as a journalist, wrote screenplays for Hollywood (including *Downhill Racer*, which starred Robert Redford) and directed films such as *Three*, with Charlotte Rampling and Sam Waterston. His third novel, *A Sport and a Pastime*, involving a passionate affair between an American man and a French woman, published in 1967, earned him international reputation. The publication of this novel, which takes its title from a Quranic verse on the essence of earthly life, marked a turning point in Salter's career and set the standard of his literary ambition and mastery.

This was followed by *Light Years, Solo Faces*, a collection of stories titled *Dusk* and his memoirs, *Burning the Days*. Between

1997 and 2000, he only published revisions of his first two novels, and in 2005, a new collection of short stories called ***Last Night***. His work has received numerous awards, including the 1989 PEN/Faulkner Award.

Context: Joining the United States Army as World War II comes to an end is a declaration of principles in a world, our world, where there is only more and more self-interest, while principles, rather than playing in the Champions League, are relegated to the Second Division. Liquid society has almost vaporised our principles.

In this world, respect is still maintained for Homer, even though we don't know it; although not everything is as simple and simplifying as seeing it in black and white. There is a suspicion that reading Salter has something binomial about it: either you enter into him or you don't. To continue with the strange Homeric example, we could say that some beings are characters who appeared in the ***Iliad*** and its endless wars. And others, less primary, perhaps evoke those of the ***Odyssey***.

Some, inexplicably to others, do not shy away from war. Others, who are smarter, more practical, and not tied to that tremendous burden of feeling that honour must be defended, whatever the cost, seek other forms of life. In a certain way, perhaps in their own way, these people try to sidestep away from this war which is so present in the world; they avoid it because fighting is tiring and, with all forms of dignity, and legitimately so, they sneak away. These people are surely smarter, perhaps even admirable, but they are not so heroic, or perhaps they are in their own way. Both types of people are necessary.

Salter would surely have been Faulkner's friend. They both understood the word honour in a similar way. He probably would have also got on well with Arturo Pérez Reverte, each of them being singularly different and powerful at the same time.

His extraordinary potency is unspoken. It is never explicit. He is not an author for fans of the ***Top Gun*** films. But his own ***Iliad*** was neither a celluloid nor a tall tale. He fought in Korea without making a big fuss about it. He wouldn't have posted it on Facebook or LinkedIn. I suspect he wouldn't have known what either platform was, even if he had been born sixty years later; Salter would probably never have had Twitter. That is also another form of his expression, which I think contains a very peculiar, rare and admirable form of greatness.

b. FRAGMENTS OF HIS WORK

"As Rilke says, there are no classes for beginners in life, the most difficult thing is always asked of one right away. Still, they are not so bad, these black men. They are very sweet, I have heard, they are very tender. They will spend every penny they have on a girl, absolutely everything. They are foolishly generous. I envy them for that."

"I felt, with him— it's difficult to explain— that he could not be challenged by lies. He had already proved he cared nothing for them. That was the whole point of his life."

"In a way I could calmly expect that from this point they would begin, having discovered all there was so soon, to lose interest in each other, to grow cold, but these acts are sometimes merely an introduction—in the great, carnal duets

I think they must often be—and I search for the exact ciphers which serve to open it all as if for a safe combination."

"Solitude. One knows instinctively it has benefits that must be more deeply satisfying than those of other conditions, but still it is difficult. And besides, how is one to distinguish between conditions which are valuable, which despite their hatefulness give us strength or impel us to great things and others we would be far better free of? Which are precious and which are not? Why is it so hard to be happy alone? Why is it impossible? Why, whenever I am idle, sometimes even before, in the midst of doing something, do I slowly but inevitably become subject to the power of their acts."

c. BRIEF COMMENTARY

Although it sounds a little outrageous and over the top, in a way, we can sometimes feel that certain people's lives could ultimately be a tragedy. A muffled existence. And I think James Salter knows this (or some of his characters at least), but neither the novelist nor his characters live on the run, terrified by this reality. His silent and forceful way of telling the truth means he can break your heart with a sentence. Without shouting it from the rooftops. It's like he is telling you in silence. In this short anthology, Salter may appear as a writer who is more attune to male readers. His female counterpart for this book would be Elena Ferrante, an author for a female audience who, I suppose, will know how to enjoy her better. And I'll say it again and again: these writers are both giants of literature.

A Sport and a Pastime makes you work to keep your balance: only twice in my life has reading made me dizzy. Dizzy with admiration. I have never read an erotic relationship described in such a powerful way, with such hypnotic elegance.

It would be very difficult to read Salter from the severity of a denial of sensual pleasure. I cannot imagine Calvino reading Salter, if they had been contemporaries. Well, I can imagine it, although in terms of the reformer immediately going to fetch logs for the fire in which to burn him alive.

When James Salter describes a couple breaking up, your universe suffers as if you were that broken couple, and also a large part of their lives which are falling apart at the seams. Salter perceives that you are more than just a spectator, watching what he describes: he makes the reader become the world, assisting – impassive and at the same time suffering – a collapse. Another one. Of two beings. From his world. Of a world, of the world.

This is why we should repeat the phrase from *The Washington Post*, "Salter is the contemporary writer most admired and envied by other writers. He can, when he wants, break your heart with a sentence."

All the same, to only read *A Sport and a Pastime* or to admire him only for this novel would be to stick with a solid but very thin layer of Salter. It is not even his most significant book. All his books are magnificent works of human knowledge. The way he describes life, love and heartbreak, war, travel, time, and farewells is astounding.

Salter is a great among the greats.

d. EVERYDAY REFLECTIONS

A house with a fire lit in winter is more inviting. It is better at keeping away the cold. To read James Salter is to light a fire in the cold of winter. It provides warmth in the midst of being alone and serene. It is like the camel-hair blanket that is offered to those who take shelter in the sanatorium of **The Magic Mountain**. It is to read, surrounded by light, lucidity, solitude and intimacy.

Strange as it may sound (since reading is in itself a lonely act), reading Salter is like reading in company.

e. OTHER RELEVANT FRAGMENTS

"At last she was willing, did not resist. The two of us were face to face, she was glimmering in the dark. That hotel no longer exists, although the act remains, that common and ordinary act that divided life in two, one part breaking apart right there and the other extending gloriously onwards."

"Early that winter, he and I went to Korea. We had eagerly read - it passed from hand to hand - the first definitive report, a sort of letter about the enemy airplanes that had suddenly appeared in the war, Russian planes, MIG-15s, and when the chance came, like men running to a claims office, we had raced to volunteer. There were two openings that month and we got them. It was not only the report, the war itself was whispering an invitation: Meet me. Whatever we were, we felt inauthentic. You were not anything unless you had fought."

"There are really only two kinds of office: those who have virtue and those without. Not that either is preferable - there are times when virtue is a terrible defect."

f. SUGGESTED READING

Burning the Days, London, Vintage, 2010.
A Sport and a Pastime, London, Picador Modern Classics, 2006.
Last Night, Barcelona, London, 2006.
All That Is, Barcelona, London, 2014.

Lucidity as a lethal mutation
Miguel Torga

a. WHO IS MIGUEL TORGA?

Miguel Torga, pseudonym of the Portuguese doctor, novelist and poet, Adolfo Correia da Rocha, was born in São Martinho de Anta in 1907 and died in Coimbra in 1995. To read his *Diary* is to see, through his privileged eyes, a large part of the history of Portugal in the 20th century, but – and this is what is really important – it is also to understand a human soul, with a truly harrowing depth, solitude, lucidity and secret tenderness. He was the first to win the Camões Prize (1989), the most important award in the Portuguese language, and equivalent to the Cervantes Prize in Spain.

Context: Portugal, at the time, is a powerful country, with a rich domestic life, and a very different sensibility from that of its Iberian neighbour. It also, like Spain, had its own dictatorship, but Portugal's, instead of being visceral and bloodthirsty, had more of a discreet *saudade* as its backbone. In Portugal they will tell you about Fernando Pessoa (1888-1935) if you ask, while in many places in Spain people get offended if you don't even know who their hairdresser is.

b. FRAGMENTS OF HIS WORK

"Coimbra, March 2, 1953. A perfect day. From nine in the morning until seven in the afternoon, I was sowing confidence! My throat began to hurt. But I have left the office with some inner comfort. The melancholic boy will react, the girl in love will get her boyfriend back, and that guy whose ears were ringing, with a little resignation and the pills I have prescribed, may not suffer so much.

It is fine to be a doctor and a poet! You can give the double of yourself. Young people come to ask me for help because I write verses; the old ones, because I prescribe medicines for them. And we all come out winning. They do because they feel that they are not alone in the world; and I, after all, do too. And I do these things, these daily actions without flashes of heroism, but usefully and modestly, as it suits my shy nature, camouflaged by the intellectual and physical violence of a compensatory nature."

"Sometimes I wonder if I could be a simple chair and table writer, a man without a commitment to flesh and blood, without this communion of tears and pus that, later on in my verses, I will try to sublimate. Every morning, when I open the door of the office, I carry two men who are in dialogue, within me. One speaks ill of destiny and the other speaks well. But when, like today, I really manage to give life a little push, when night comes, they both bring it to a close, reconciled."

c. BRIEF COMMENTARY

Many of us will agree that the two most beautiful professions in the world are those of a doctor and teacher. Torga, being a poet and a doctor, is somehow an example of both (since as a poet and author, he also teaches). As another great writer, João Guimarães Rosa (1908-1967), put it,

> *"The master is not the one who teaches;*
> *it's the one who suddenly learns."*

Torga shows the essential humility of good things.

d. EVERYDAY REFLECTIONS

Running away from the bombast is beautiful. Having meaning, a commitment to duty, to your profession, to loving your vocation… these are gifts in life that we have surely worked for and deserved.

In short, you have to fight for what is worthwhile.

e. OTHER RELEVANT FRAGMENTS

> *"While you do not reach, do not rest, of no future you want only half."*

> *"Porto, November 14, 1957. Here is the world, again! And how beautiful it is, the scoundrel! It is full of sun, flowers, noise, and, most importantly, it does not smell like medicine. It also jabs us from time to time, obviously, but they are no longer jabs of morphine. They are injections of life, of love. Or*

they seem so to me…"

f. SUGGESTED READING

Diário II (1987-1993), ('Diary II'), unavailable in English.
Tales from the Mountain, Manchester, Carcanet Press Ltd., 1995.
Orfeu Rebelde, (Rebel Orpheus), unavailable in English.
Diário (1932-1987), (Diary) unavailable in English.
The Creation of the World, Manchester, Carcanet Press Ltd.,
1996.

The poet illuminated
with immensity
Giuseppe Ungaretti

Giuseppe Ungaretti, a poet considered to be part of the Hermetic group (along with Montale, Quasimodo, Luzi and Campana), was also a teacher and translator. He was born in Alexandria, Egypt, in 1888, and died in Milan in 1970. His family, who were Italian and from Lucca, had moved to Egypt because his father, who died a year after Giuseppe was born, was working on the construction of the Suez Canal. In 1912 he moved to study at the Sorbonne in Paris. He worked on *Lacerba* magazine with Giovani Papini, and this is where his first poems appeared. In Paris he lived an intense intellectual life, he had dealings with the philosopher Henri Bergson and became friends with Philippe Jaccottet, who translated his work into French. He also met Picasso, Leger, De Chirico, Braque, Apollinaire, Cendrars, Satie and Juan Gris among others. In 1913 his great friend Moammed Sceab committed suicide, to whom he dedicated one of his greatest poems. In 1914 he returned to Italy and, when World War I broke out, he volunteered in 1915. He fought in Carso (province of Trieste) and then in France.

In 1916 he published in Italian the collection of poems *The Sunken Keep*, where he reflects his experiences of the war, among them the impressive *"Vigil"*. In 1919 he settled in Paris, married Jeanne Dupoix, and published a second collection of poems entitled *Allegria*.

After the war, in which he felt he was part of the "docile fibre of the universe," he worked for a time at the Italian embassy in Paris. He regularly collaborated with magazines and later worked in a ministry as a language teacher. In 1933 he published *The Feeling of Time*. Between 1936 and 1942 he was a professor of Italian at the University of São Paulo in Brazil. It was a period during which, in 1939, he lost his second son, Antonietto, who died at the age of nine. It was an experience that permeated part of his verses in the book *The Pain*, a work of astonishing tenderness and desolation. In 1942, the year in which he was appointed academic, he took up a permanent position as professor at the University of Rome, a position he held until 1958.

Life of a man is the work that gathers together all his poetry. He died in Milan on June 2, 1970.

Context: To be born far from the land of your mother tongue is a form of exile. To discover poetry at sixteen is a way of establishing an internal, intimate country. To arrive in Paris at the age of twenty-eight in 1916 is to open yourself up to a great world. And to volunteer in the First World War is to understand pain.

Not everyone has this form of contact with the reality of life, nor the opportunity to be with people who are geniuses of the twentieth century. Not everyone has lived in several countries either (Erasmus scholarships did not appear until 1987. Let's not forget that then travelling was something much more unique, rare and important than it is nowadays). Nor has everyone resided (or resisted) on other continents. And very few, luckily – yet any at all is too many – have lost a child.

Not all human beings reach this intensity or have these types of experiences. Not all of us can create, from every key person in our life, a fertile ground for a poem which is yet to be written.

Ungaretti is much more than all this. Much more than a cosmopolitan culture and vital nomadism. Ungaretti is more than life, the Earth, tenderness, knowledge and pain.

Ungaretti is the poet of the ***Life of a man***.

b. FRAGMENTS OF HIS WORK

Eternal*
Between one flower picked and the other given
the inexpressible nothing.

In memory**
(Locvizza, 30 September 1910)

---

* **Eterno** / *Tra un fiore colto e l'altro donato / l'inesprimibile nulla.*
** **In memoria** (Locvizza, il 30 septtembre de 1910) / *Si chiamava / **Moammed Sceab** / /*
Discendente / di emiri di nomadi / suicida / perché non aveva più / Patria / Amò la Francia / e mutò nome / / Fu Marcel / ma non era Francese / e non sapeva più / vivere / nella tenda dei suoi / dove si ascolta la cantilena / del Corano / gustando un caffè / / E non sapeva / sciogliere / il canto / del suo abbandono / / L'ho accompagnato / insieme alla padrona dell'albergo / dove abitavamo / a Parigi / dal numero 5 della rue des Carmes / appassito vicolo in discesa. / / Riposa / nel camposanto d'Ivry / sobborgo che pare / sempre / in una giornata / di una / decomposta fiera / / E forse io solo / so ancora / che visse.

His name was
Mohammed Sceab.

Descendant
of emirs of nomads

a suicide
because he had no homeland
left
He loved France
and changed his name.

He was Marcel
but wasn't French
and no longer knew
how to live
in his people's tent
where you hear the Koran
being chanted
while you savour your coffee
And he didn't know how
to set free
the song
of his desolation.

I went with him
and the proprietress of the hotel
where we lived in Paris
from number 5 Rue des Carmes
an old faded alley sloping downhill.

He rests
in the graveyard at Ivry
a suburb that always
seems
like the day
a fair breaks down.
And perhaps only I
still know
he lived.

Vigil*
(Summit four, 23 December 1915)

An entire night long
Crouched close
To a companion
Slaughtered
Mouth
Clenched
Up at the full moon
With the congestion
Of his hands
Thrust
Into my silence
I have written
Letters full of love.

---

* **Veglia** / *Un'intera nottata / buttato vicino / a un compagno / massacrato / con la sua boc-*
ca / digrignata / volta al plenilunio, / con la congestione / delle sue mani / penetrata /
nel mio silenzio / ho scritto / lettere piene d'amore. / Non sono mai stato / tanto / attaccato
alla vita.

I have never held
So
Hard to life.

c. BRIEF COMMENTARY

What is poetry, among many other things, if not the condensed expression of our need for meaning and love, our will to exist, our need for art as a form of expression and transcendence? What is the apparently useless for? Why create? Why look for ways that help give voice to feelings or thoughts that perhaps, in the best of cases, we had already sensed? Reading poetry is a vessel that can be reached. There is no need to study for a boat license. It is enough just to dare to get on the ship and set sail. And go out to sea, be it coasting or to more open waters. It does not matter.

Start reading poetry and give in to it. Read it and focus on the amazement. The admiration. The emotion. The respect. The surprise. The anger. The joy. The bewilderment. The pain. The compassion. The surrender. All these feelings and thoughts fit into Ungaretti. It is like reading something that permeates our life. It is like reading poems that begin to filter a porous rock; your life contains the very essence of living. A universe of life and sensitivity begin to trickle down, in the most astounding way. Reading poetry is many things. It is what each of us wants it to be. Reading poetry demands dedication. Go in naked, come out more naked, yet at the same time much more equipped to live, and die.

To read Ungaretti is to immerse yourself in great poetry. Poetry born out of loss: his father, whom he does not know, a son, a native landscape. It is the loss of the war; it is that of exile… It is losing the possibility of seeing his son grow up, of seeing him reach a full life.

Through despair, the poet discovers human responsibility and the fragility of his ambitions. Ungaretti, amid the pessimism with which he contemplates the tragic human condition, finds a message of hope for mankind. In a more intimate way, we can see that reading Ungaretti is to grasp the land from which we came and to which we will return. It is having our hands soaked with our own being. To focus on what we have a right to feel. To give us access to the best and most intimate versions of ourselves. To read Ungaretti is, in his own words, "to illuminate oneself with immensity."

d. EVERYDAY REFLECTIONS

We cannot live without poetry. We do. But it is like living with a part of you missing, without that essential dimension necessary for every human being. Luckily, we collect, in a more or less tacit or explicit way, small scraps of poetry through every great work of art. The everyday also offers us a poetic experience. But you have to open your eyes to it, in a generous way, being open to the beautiful.

It's like going to sea for the first time. If you have a snorkel and a mask, you can immerse yourself in a reality which is powerful, far from the surface of the water. Life is much more intense, rich and complete. You start to look towards the bottom, beneath the skin of the sea.

e. OTHER RELEVANT FRAGMENTS

Saint Martin of Carso*
(Valloncello dell'Albero Isolato, 27 August 1916)

*Of these homes
Nothing is left
But the rare
Shred of wall
Of the many
Whom I once met
Nothing is left
Nothing much at all*

*But in my heart
No cross is lacking*

*For my heart is
the most shattered land of all.*

* **San Martino del Carso** / *(Valloncello dell'Albero Isolato, 27 de agosto de 1916)* /
*Di queste case / non è rimasto / che qualche / brandello di muro / / Di tanti / che mi corris-
pondevano / non è rimasto / neppure tanto / / Ma nel cuore / nessuna croce manca / / è il mio
cuore / il paese più straziato.*

186

Lucca*

At my house, in Egypt, after dinner, the rosary said,
my mother would tell us of these places.
My childhood was filled with their wonder.
The city has a God-fearing and fanatical traffic.
Within these walls one stays only temporary;
Here the goal is to leave.
I sat down outside, at the entrance of the tavern, with people
Who speak to me of California as one of their farms.
With terror I discover the features of these people.
Now I feel it flow, hot in my veins, the blood of my dead.
I took a scythe.
I have fallen into the strong smell of my land.
Farewell, desires and nostalgias,
I know of the past and the future as much as it is given to a
man to know.
There remains to me nothing unknown, not even my origin
and my destiny.
There is left to me nothing more to profane or bemoan.
I have enjoyed and suffered everything;
And nothing is left for me but to resign myself to death.
Which is to raise a child quietly.

---

* **Lucca** / *A casa mia, in Egitto, dopo cena, recitato il rosario, mia madre / ci parlava di questi posti. / La mia infanzia ne fu tutta meravigliata. / La città ha un traffico timorato e fanatico. / In queste mura non ci si sta che di passaggio. / Qui la meta è partire. / Mi sono seduto al fresco sulla porta dell'osteria con della gente / che mi parla di California come d'un suo podere. / Mi scopro con terrore nei connotati di queste persone. / Ora lo sento scorrere caldo nelle mie vene, il sangue dei miei morti. / Ho preso anch'io una zappa. / Nelle cosce fumanti della terra mi scopro a ridere. / Addio desideri, nostalgie. / So di passato e d'avvenire quanto un uomo può saperne. / Conosco ormai il mio destino, e la mia origine. / Non mi rimane che rassegnarmi a morire. / Alleverò dunque tranquillamente una prole. / Quando un appetito maligno mi spingeva negli amori mortali, lodavo / la vita. / Ora che considero, anch'io, l'amore come una garanzia della specie, / ho in vista la morte.*

When a malevolent appetite spurred me to amours to
annihilate me, I praised life;
But now that I too consider love as a guarantee of the species,
I have death in my view.

Soldiers*

We are as
in autumn
on branches
the leaves.

f. SUGGESTED READING

Allegria, New York, Archipelago, 2020.
Sentimento del tempo. La terra promessa (Feeling of Time. The Promised Land), unavailable in English.
Il dolore (Pain), unavailable in English.
Il taccuino del vecchio (The Old Man's Notebook), unavailable in English.
Life of a Man, Montblanc, Hamish Hamilton Ltd., 1958.

---

* **Soldados** / *Si sta come* / *d'autunno* / *sugli alberi* / *le foglie.*

The infinite pleasure of reading (and the fortune of being a reader)
Irene Vallejo

She was born in 1979 in Zaragoza. She studied Classical Philology and obtained a European doctorate from the universities of Zaragoza and Florence. She writes a weekly column in the *Heraldo de Aragón*. In both her journalistic collaborations and investigations, and in her fields of research, she analyses the relevance of the ancient world.

She has published two compilations of her weekly columns, *El pasado que te espera* ('The Past That Awaits You') and *Alguien habló de nosotros* ('Someone Spoke of Us').

She has two published novels, *La luz sepultada* ('The Buried Light') and *El silbido del arquero* ('The Archer's Whistle'). The latter is a story of adventure and love, set in a legendary age, but which reflects contemporary conflicts. She has also cultivated children's and youth literature with the works *El inventor de viajes*, ('The Inventor of Journeys') illustrated by José Luis Cano, and *La leyenda de las mareas mansas* ('The Legend of the Gentle Tides'), in collaboration with the painter Lina Vila.

El infinito en un junco ('Infinity in a Reed') is her masterpiece. She has received the following awards: The Narrative Critical Eye Award 2019, The Libraries Recommend Non-Fiction Award 2020, and the Owl Award for Best Book of 2019, awarded by the Aragonese Association of Friends of the Book.

Context: Irene Vallejo has perfectly demonstrated the accuracy of Nuccio Ordine's thesis on the usefulness of the useless. In a screen-obsessed world which is often responsible for destroying our serenity and the pleasure we find in slowness, this wonderful author has found a direct line to the obvious relevance of the ancient world and, by extension, to the world of books and many of the things they do to make life worth living. Kant distinguished between what has a price, and what has dignity. Irene Vallejo illustrates it on every page of *Infinity in a Reed*.

Let's move from Kant onto more practical matters: people who don't know what the humanities are for should read this book, and if they don't understand it, they should set about fixing this, perhaps with something much deeper than a mindfulness course.

If they feel it's taking forever, they need to find a way to focus, perhaps with something which can help them do a digital detox. And, finally, if this privacy fails to get them excited, and doesn't result in an intoxicating feeling of gratitude towards books, the unfortunate reader has an acute attack of indifference that, short of being fatal to the body, will be for a good part of the soul. Note: he who does not have something similar to a soul, should not even try to read this book: they will not understand anything.

b. FRAGMENTS OF HER WORK

"Mysterious groups of men on horseback travel the roads of Greece. The peasants watch them distrustfully from their land or from the entrance to their huts. Experience has taught them that only dangerous people travel: soldiers, mercenaries and slave traders. They frown and grunt until they see them sinking back over the horizon. They do not like armed outsiders. The horsemen ride without noticing the villagers. For months they have climbed mountains, they have passed over gorges, they have crossed valleys, they have waded through rivers, they have sailed from island to island. Their muscles and stamina have hardened since they were charged with this strange mission. To fulfil their task they must venture through the violent territories of a world at almost constant war. They are hunters in search of prey of a very special kind. Silent, cunning prey that leaves no footprint or trace. If these restless messengers sat in some port tavern, drinking wine, eating roasted octopus, talking and getting drunk with strangers (they never can out of caution), they could tell great stories of their journeys. They have entered plague-ridden lands. They have traversed regions ravaged by fires, they have looked upon the hot ash of destruction and the brutality of rebels and mercenaries on the warpath. As maps of vast regions do not yet exist, they have become lost and wandered aimlessly for days under the fury of the sun or storms. They have had to drink revolting

water that has caused hideous diarrhoea. Whenever it rains, the mules and carts get stuck in the puddles; between screams and cursing they have dragged them to their knees and until they kiss the mud. When nightfall catches them far from any shelter, only their cloak protects them from scorpions. They have known the maddening torment of lice and the constant fear of bandits that invade the roads. Many times, riding through vast solitudes, their blood runs cold as they imagine a group of bandits waiting for them, holding their breath, hiding at some bend in the road to pounce on them, kill them in cold blood, steal their bags and leave their warm corpses strewn among the bushes. It is understandable that they are afraid. The king of Egypt has entrusted them with large sums of money before sending them to carry out his orders at the other end of the coast. At that time, just a few decades after Alexander's death, travelling with a large fortune was very risky, almost suicidal. And although the daggers of thieves, contagious diseases and shipwrecks threaten to derail such an expensive mission, the pharaoh insists on sending his agents from the country of the Nile, across borders and great distances, in all directions. He passionately desires, with impatience and an aching thirst for possession, that prey that his secret hunters track down for him, facing unknown dangers. The prying peasants who sit at the door of their huts, the mercenaries and the bandits would have opened their eyes in amazement and their mouths in disbelief if they had known what the foreign horsemen were after. Books, they were looking for books. It was the best kept secret of the Egyptian court. The Lord of the Two Lands, one of the most powerful men of the time, would give his life (that of others, of course; it is always like that with kings) to get all the books in the world for his Great Library of Alexandria. He was pursuing the dream of an absolute and perfect library, the collection where all the works of all authors since the beginning of time would be gathered."

c. BRIEF COMMENTARY

If someone thinks that Homer has nothing to do with them, they are probably right. However, without suggesting that I'm better than whoever thinks like that, I do feel a certain pity towards them (and, to avoid sounding supercilious, towards myself as well, when I didn't think Homer had much to do with me either.)

You can live perfectly well without reading Homer. And you can even succeed in your professional life only knowing who Homer Simpson is. But while Simpson is also a cool guy, the author of the ***Iliad*** and the ***Odyssey*** can touch our essence as humans in a way that I tend to feel can only be achieved by those who choose to try to be chosen – yes, whoever wants to know, knows: with a lot of work done on themselves.

Irene Vallejo knows this, and she has written one of the most beautiful pieces I have ever read about books. It is about the birth of the desire to apprehend what one knows and, once captured, be a spectator of the movement that changed history: writing and the birth of the book. In Eco's words, "The book is like the spoon, scissors, the hammer, the wheel. Once invented, it cannot be improved. The book has stood the test of time… Its components may evolve, its pages may no longer be paper, but it will remain what it is."

If all this is not enough to convince you of the beauty of the books, you have to complain to the school where you sat your senior school exams, or, perhaps more accurately, have a serious conversation with the family you were lucky enough to be born into. It is useful to try to understand what happened (or, rather, what didn't happen). If one does not love any form of culture having grown up in a more or less normal world, then they must ask themselves what happened in their school and their home life. One of the two (if not both) has failed.

This book is one of the most masterful declarations of love to the book that I have read in years. It is an essential object to becoming the best version of yourself, the one to which you should always aspire to be.

I do not remember ever having read a work in which the presence of Antiquity was made evident with such elegant erudition.

d. EVERYDAY REFLECTIONS

This is not a good time for Humanism. Yet at the same time, the miasmas of fanaticism, ignorance, and contempt for the other require works like this: a book that validates, each time it is read, the enormous relevance and need for knowledge that was delivered to us by the best that have come before us. Those giants of history on whose shoulders we stand – an expression attributed to Newton, even though it already existed – to be able to continue advancing.

THIS SEASON'S LITERARY REVELATION

"Smoke, stone, clay, silk, leather, trees, plastic and light…
A journey through the life of the book and of those who
have safeguarded it for almost thirty centuries."

*"Very well written, with genuinely remarkable pages; a love
for books and reading is the atmosphere in which the pages
of this masterpiece unfold. I am absolutely sure that it will
continue to be read when its current readers are already in
the afterlife."*
MARIO VARGAS LLOSA

*"Vallejo has wisely decided to free herself from an academic style
and has opted for the voice of the storyteller. History is understood
not as a string of cited documents, but as a fable. Thus, for the
common reader (whom Virginia Woolf defended) this charming
essay is more moving and more immediate, because it is simply a
tribute to the book, made on behalf of a passionate reader."*
ALBERTO MANGUEL, "Babelia", *El País*

*"Those books that temper you, that pacify you, that impose
a rhythm of reading on you, that calm your nerves, are not
usually found, despite their necessity, in the first lines few of a
latest release. The last of these books that I have discovered is
entitled **Infinity in a Reed** and is by Irene Vallejo."*
JUAN JOSÉ MILLÁS, *El País*

"You can be a master philologist and at the same time write like the angels. Irene Vallejo gilds the lily of communication until she turns the dialogue she has with the reader into a literary celebration."
LUIS ALBERTO DE CUENCA, *ABC*

"An admirable examination of the origins of the greatest instrument of freedom that human beings have given themselves: the book."
RAFAEL ARGULLOL

"Irene Vallejo's books, which are clear and intelligent, read so well and invite you to think. In the best humanistic line."
CARLOS GARCÍA GUAL

"A very free and very wise and very digressive journey through the world of books, from the creation of the Library of Alexandria until the fall of the Roman Empire; Irene Vallejo has just written a wonderful, universal, unique book."
JORDI CARRIÓN, *The New York Times*

e. OTHER RELEVANT FRAGMENTS

"This individual freedom, yours, is a conquest of independent thought versus protected thought, and has been achieved step by step over time."

"[...] here an attractive paradox is hidden: that we can all love the past is a profoundly revolutionary fact."

"In a covered gallery he says he has seen the sacred library on which was written "Place of Care for the soul".

"From Anatolia to the gates of India, in the expanded and mestizo Hellenistic world, being Greek was no longer a matter of birth or genetics; it had much more to do with loving the Homeric poems."

"[…] we prefer to ignore that progress and beauty include pain and violence."

"Ulysses is a struggling and shaken creature who prefers authentic sadness to artificial happiness."

f. SUGGESTED READING

El infinito en un junco (Infinity in a Reed), unavailable in English. Madrid, Siruela, 2020.

Reading it will make some women – and many, many brave and generous men – better understand what it is to be a woman

Virginia Woolf

a. WHO IS VIRGINIA WOOLF?

Virginia Woolf (1882-1941) grew up and lived in a privileged environment, surrounded by writers, artists and intellectuals.

However, her life was not easy. Her parents believed, as was customary at the time, that women should not be educated outside the home. Although they sent their sons to Cambridge University, they educated their daughters themselves, and also gave them free access to a very well stocked library. It did not occur to them that Virginia could work; on the other hand, they considered it appropriate and not at odds with her status as a woman for her to write.

Her childhood was marked by frequent visits of many family friends, important figures in the artistic life of the time (Thackeray, Henry James, Thomas Hardy, Alfred Tennyson, Edward Burne-Jones…), her trips to the Cornish seaside –

portrayed in many of her works – but also by her bouts of depression, some experienced when she was very young.

She was deeply affected by the death of her mother (1895) and that of her stepsister, who had taken on the role of her mother. During those years, she and her sister Vanessa were abused by a stepbrother and a cousin, and when her father died in 1905, Virginia had already attempted suicide for the first time.

When her father died, she and her siblings, Adrian and Vanessa, sold the family home and moved to the Bloomsbury area of London. This new house became the meeting place for her older brother's friends, a meeting that became known as the "Bloomsbury Group", made up of intellectuals such as the writer E. M. Forster, the economist J. M. Keynes and the philosophers Bertrand Russell and Ludwig Wittgenstein.

In 1912 she married Leonard Woolf for love, with whom she founded the Hogarth publishing house, where much of her work was published. However, her recurring episodes of depression led her to suicide, and she drowned herself in the river, her coat pockets full of stones.

It has been said that one of the main characteristics of her writing was the enriching presence of emotions and everyday situations, of which little was said in those days. Another of her contributions to the modern-day novel was her use of the interior monologue and the stream of consciousness, which gave depth to the construction of her characters.

She was an inspiration for the liberal feminist suffragist movement and great authors, such as Simone de Beauvoir, especially for her analysis of the use of violence by men against women to repress them politically and intellectually.

She also stressed the need to be financially independent and was a pioneer in speaking of the ghost of the "perfect woman": the one who can solve any problem, is always smiling, knows how to cook, sing and do embroidery. In order to write and be famous, she had to fight against that "angel of the house," and she questioned what it is to be a woman. Woolf wrote and published on these subjects at a time when the hegemony of men, in all fields, went unchallenged.

Context: Woolf lived in between two centuries, with the First World War and the Russian Revolution as crucial events, which, with their immense cruelty, destabilised the way of understanding the world and changed the political and economic map. However, the causes of a new global confrontation were being forged nearby. Even if you lived in highly civilised England, it would not have been easy to escape the enormous unrest happening at that moment in history.

b. FRAGMENTS OF HER WORK

"A woman must have money and a room of her own if she is to write fiction; and that, as you will see, leaves the great problem of the true nature of woman and the true nature of fiction unsolved."

"Indeed, if woman had no existence save in the fiction written by men, one would imagine her a person of the utmost importance; very various; heroic and mean; splendid and sordid; infinitely beautiful and hideous in the extreme; as great as a man, some think even greatest.

But this is woman in fiction. In fact, as Professor Trevelyan points out, she was locked up, beaten and flung about the room. A very queer, composite being thus emerges. Imaginatively she is of the highest importance; practically she is completely insignificant. She pervades poetry from cover to cover; she is all but absent from history. She dominates the lives of kings and conquerors in fiction; in fact she was the slave of any boy whose parents forced a ring upon her finger. Some of the most inspired words, some of the most profound thoughts in literature fall from her lips; in real life she could hardly read, could scarcely spell, and was the property of her husband."

c. BRIEF COMMENTARY

A Room of One's Own, a crucial book in the history of feminism, written in a style that mixes evocation, irritation and irony, details the material conditions that limit women's access to writing.

It explains that women cannot travel alone to open their spirit, they cannot sit alone on the terrace of a restaurant to think or access the university library (where they can only enter accompanied by a teacher or a member of the university).

It also speaks of the obligations derived from marriage, from children, which leave little time for women to read or write. After the exclamations of an old clergyman, who asserted that no woman can have the genius of Shakespeare, Woolf performs an interesting exercise in explaining the impediments of all kinds that one of Shakespeare's sisters would have had to endure in order to write. She would not, in fact, have succeeded.

One of the basic ideas of the book is the insistence that the female artist must have financial independence and an intimate space to work. Let us remember that women did not have the right to control the money they earned; it was left to their husbands.

Woolf declares that, having obtained the right to vote a few years before, she considers it more important to control her own money than to be able to vote. "Give her a room of her own and five hundred a year, let her speak her mind and leave out half that she now puts in, and she will write a better book one of these days."

What did five hundred pounds represent in those days? A CPI updater indicates that it would be equivalent to 34,000 euros in 2018.

d. EVERYDAY REFLECTIONS

There is still a glaring inequality between men and women today. Almost a century after Virginia Woolf's denunciations, there are still gender injustices which are yet to be resolved. It is clear that laws are not enough (even if they are necessary) to help educate us in this new reality that must lead to a change in people's mentalities. That is why it is highly recommended to read the authors who have reflected the most on the subject, and to let their message sink into us deeply.

Virginia Woolf was a woman, but above all, she was also a great artist. She suffered from the constant antagonism of society against her creative desires. An intelligent woman of a certain social status, she knew how to avoid obstacles and left us a work of unparalleled quality. But, like her, let us think about what it takes to unleash creativity: a space of peace, a time of solitude, a means to survive.

e. OTHER RELEVANT FRAGMENTS

"It is obvious that the values of women differ very often from the values which have been made by the other sex; naturally, this is so. Yet it is the masculine values that prevail."

"Yet who reads to bring about an end, however desirable? Are there not some pursuits that we practise because they are good in themselves, and some pleasures that are final? And is not this among them? I have sometimes dreamt, at least, that when the Day of Judgment dawns and the great conquerors and lawyers and statesmen come to receive their rewards—their crowns, their laurels, their names carved indelibly upon imperishable marble—the Almighty will turn to Peter and will say, not without a certain envy when he sees us coming with our books under our arms, "Look, these need no reward. We have nothing to give them here. They have loved reading."

"There is no gate, no lock, no bolt that you can set upon the freedom of my mind."

f. SUGGESTED READING

A Room of One's Own, London, Penguin Books, 2019.
The Waves, London, Random House, 2016.
Mrs. Dalloway, London, Penguin Books, 2018.

Learning that there is more than one wisdom
Marguerite Yourcenar

a. WHO IS MARGUERITE YOURCENAR?

Marguerite Yourcenar, novelist, poet, playwright and French-language translator, was born in Brussels in 1903, although she became a US citizen in 1947. She died in Maine, United States, in 1987. Her father, an aristocrat, took care of her education, since her mother passed away when she was only ten days old. Despite not having attended school, she was the first woman to enter the French Academy, and in 1986 she received the Legion of Honour. Her literature is highly influenced by André Gide (1869-1951), Romain Rolland (1866-1944) and Constantin Kavafis (1863-1933). She travelled the world out of curiosity until she settled in the United States in the early 1950s. She lived with her partner, Grace Frick, until her death. Her book, *Memoirs of Hadrian*, is one of the great works of the 20th century.

Context: Yourcenar is an aristocrat in the etymological sense of the word. She had an elite education. She was taught through placing the most exquisite culture you can think of at the centre. She lived through the century with the lucidity of cosmopolitanism and enjoyed a free life both in spirit and in practice. The axes of her life were marked by the education given to her by her father, Europe, polyglotism, humanist culture, the Eastern world and the United States.

b. FRAGMENTS OF HER WORK

"It is not that I despise men. If I did I should have no right, and no reason, to try to govern. I know them to be vain, ignorant, greedy, and timorous, capable of almost anything for the sake of success, or for raising themselves in esteem (even in their own eyes), or simply for avoidance of suffering. I know, for I am like them, at least from time to time, or could have been. Between another and myself the differences which I can recognize are too slight to count for much in the final total; I try therefore to maintain a position as far removed from the cold superiority of the philosopher as from the arrogance of a ruling Caesar. The most benighted of men are not without some glimmerings of the divine: that murderer plays passing well upon the flute; this overseer flaying the backs of his slaves is perhaps a dutiful son; this simpleton would share with me his last piece of bread. And there are few who cannot be made to learn at least something reasonably well. Our great mistake is to try to exact from each person virtues which he does not possess, and to neglect the cultivation of those which he has. I might apply here to the search for these partial virtues what I was saying earlier, in sensuous terms, about the search for beauty. I have known men infinitely nobler and more perfect than myself, like your father Antoninus, and have come across many a hero, and even a few sages. In most men I

have found little consistency in adhering to the good, but no steadier adherence to evil; their mistrust and indifference, usually more or less hostile, gave way almost too soon, almost in shame, changing too readily into gratitude and respect, which in turn were equally short-lived; even their selfishness could be bent to useful ends. I am always surprised that so few have hated me; I have had only one or two bitter enemies, for whom I was, as is always the case, in part responsible. Some few have loved me: they have given me far more that I had the right to demand, or to hope for: their deaths, and sometimes their lives. And the god whom they bear within them is often revealed when they die."

c. BRIEF COMMENTARY

Memoirs of Hadrian is written as a long letter that the emperor addresses to his adoptive grandson and future successor, Marcus Aurelius.

Hadrian explains his past, his achievements, his triumphs, the heartaches and the lessons of life, even his love for Antinous and all his philosophy.

To place the tension of this historical epoch in context, Yourcenar explains that there was a time in human history when the ancient pantheon barely existed, and the message of Jesus Christ had not yet been consolidated.

The author places the life of Hadrian in this context, a masterpiece of understanding the human condition. The almost absolute power speaks with insight, wisdom, love and an elegiac sadness of the world, of humans and of the laws that unite them in pleasure and pain.

d. EVERYDAY REFLECTIONS

Yourcenar is a compendium of human wisdom and splendour. The power of her ideas, her images and her prose does not hide the enormous lucidity of her vision.

Nothing human is alien to her, as Terence (2nd century BC) pointed out. Therefore, reading Yourcenar is an opportunity to learn the complexity and beauty of human nature.

e. OTHER RELEVANT FRAGMENTS

> *"You scarcely care for me; your filial affection goes more toward Antoninus; in me you discern a kind of wisdom which is contrary to what your masters teach you, and in my abandonment to the life of the senses you see a mode of life opposed to the severity of your own, but which nevertheless is parallel to it. Never mind: it is not necessary that you should understand me. There is more than one kind of wisdom, and all are essential in the world; it is no bad thing that they should alternate."*

f. SUGGESTED READING

Coupe de Grâce, New York, Farrar, Straus and Giroux, 1981.
Memoirs of Hadrian, New York, Farrar, Straus and Giroux, 2005.
La voix des choses, ('The Voice of Things') unavailable in English.
Alexis, New York, Farrar, Straus and Giroux, 1984.
The Abyss, New York, Farrar, Straus and Giroux, 1982.

To think about what we do with our lives, understanding our emotions and beliefs

Theodore Zeldin

a. WHO IS THEODORE ZELDIN?

Theodore Zeldin, born in Palestine under British mandate in 1933, is a philosopher, sociologist, historian and writer. He is president of the Oxford Muse Foundation. His family, of Jewish origin, left Russia to settle in Palestine, then moved to Egypt and finally settled in the United Kingdom. He graduated at the age of seventeen in Philosophy and History from the University of London (Birkbeck College) and later, already at Oxford, graduated in Modern History from Christ Church college. In both cases with the highest degree class. He later received his doctorate from St. Anthony's College, of which he was dean for thirteen years, during which time he internationalised it. Zeldin has been elected a Fellow of the British Academy and the Royal Literature Society, as well as a Fellow of the European Academy. He has been decorated as Commander of the Order of the British Empire, Commander of the Legion of Honour and Commander of the French Order of Arts and Letters, and was awarded the United

Kingdom's Wolfson History Prize. He lives in Oxford with his wife, Deirdre Wilson.

A renowned historian of France, he is internationally famous for being the author of *A History of French Passions and An Intimate History of Humanity*, published in 1994. Zeldin has said in press interviews that France has been his "laboratory", and that its citizens his "guinea pigs," whom he could investigate thanks to his rich literature and long tradition of articulation of thought. The French, with their passion for freedom of thought and free debate, provide a fruitful introduction to the complexity of existence. By studying life, and with it many of its problems, Zeldin also knows how to make us see the delights of being alive.

In his works, which are always very personal, Zeldin examines the ambitions and frustrations, the intellectual and imaginative life, the tastes and prejudices of a large group of people and connects them with moments in history, combining macro and micro-history. The Oxford Muse Foundation was formed by Zeldin in 2001. It describes its goals as "pioneering new methods to improve personal, professional and intercultural relationships in ways that satisfy both private and public values." One of his main projects is the Muse Portrait Database, which replicates Zeldin's keen interest in people and the richness they contain. Individuals are free to submit their own self-portraits, including whatever they want the world to know about them.

The Oxford muse claims that people can be helped "to clarify their tastes, attitudes and goals in many different aspects of life; and to sum up the conclusions they have drawn from their experiences in their own words."

A selection of these portraits can be found in the **Guide to an Unknown City** (2004), which contains the writings of a wide variety of Oxford residents. Similarly, the **Guide to an Unknown University** (2006) allowed professors, students, alumni, administrators, and maintenance staff to reveal what they normally do not tell each other.

In 2007, Zeldin was appointed to a committee advising the French government of Nicolas Sarkozy on labour market reforms.

Context: Being born into a family that fled from White Russia, and arrived in Palestine, is a relevant and unique starting point. His father, a road and bridge engineer, who was also a colonel in the Tsar's Army and a socialist – although he did not like the Bolsheviks – did not like either the Zionism he saw in Palestine or the Arab nationalism that they experienced in Egypt, so the family moved permanently to the United Kingdom.

Perhaps this cosmopolitanism, imposed by life and adopted as a genuine form of curiosity and generosity in his way of listening, have given him an enormous capacity to understand the other, in a different but common way to Kapuscinski, another genius of human thought.

Zeldin is a wise man who listens. He is a patient person with an orderly mind, with an enormous empathy towards the other that allows him to learn and understand the mechanisms of emotions and beliefs, which limit or enable our actions and the paths taken by each of our decisions.

To cross paths with Zeldin is to add to our lives a deep, close, curious, sincere, open and generous perspective towards such powerful subjects as the French and their passions, history, happiness, conversation, intimacy, the future of work and gastronomy, among others.

b. FRAGMENTS OF HIS WORK

"The consumer society is a giant tranquiliser for raw nerves."

"Behind Juliette's misfortunes, I see all those who have lived but thought of themselves as failures, or been treated as such. The worst sense of failure was to realise that one had not really lived at all, not been seen as an independent human being, never been listened to, never been asked for an opinion, regarded as a chattel, the property of another. That was what happened publicly to slaves. We are all of us descended from slaves, or almost slaves."

"I start with the present and work backwards, just as I start with the personal and move to the universal. Whenever I have come across an impasse in present-day ambitions, as revealed in the case studies of people I have met, I have sought a way out by balancing them against a background of all human experience in all centuries, asking how they might have behaved if, instead of relying only their own memories, they had been able to use those of the whole of humanity."

"Enough is known, enough has been written, about what divides people; my purpose is to investigate what they have in common."

"Today hope is sustained above all by the prospect of meeting new people."

"[Lisa] complains that they assume experiences nurses like herself will just go on doing their duty, earning little more than young nurses straight out of school: she wants recognition of her experience, not necessarily in money, but in respect. The lack of it has turned everything sour. [...] nobody forsaw the world shortage of respect."

"Why, after centuries of experience, are humans still so awkward, rude, inattentive in conversation, with even 40 per cent of Americans – brought up to regard silence as unfriendly – complaining that they are too shy to speak freely? The answer is that conversation is still in its infancy."

"Deborah Tannen, after a lifetime of research, concludes that they cannot understand each other, that they mean quite different things when they speak, that women want comfort from those they converse with, while mean seek solutions to problems. [...] Only when people learn to converse will they begin to be equal."

"One may feel isolated in one's own town, but one has forebearers all over the world."

"More and more people are becoming abnormal, and are not fitting neatly into a single civilisation."

"Marco Polo has such curiosity that he forgets fear."

"In any life there is an element of victory over fear, which needs to be searched for, though it may be a false victory. Again and again, apparently intelligent people ooze contempt to protect themselves from they cannot understand, as animals defend their territories with foul smells."

c. BRIEF COMMENTARY

History of the Intimate Life of Humanity is a magnificent book, examining the personal concerns of people in many different civilisations, both past and present. It is a continuous crossover of history and the stories of individual people. It sheds light on the way emotions, curiosities, relationships, and fears have evolved through the centuries, and how they could have evolved differently.

In it we discover some of the issues that affect us, and which are of most interest today: freedom, tolerance, sex, loneliness, power, work, eating…

Based on specific cases, Zeldin reveals a network of surprising affinities between human beings from very different times and places; relationships with the past whose knowledge conditions our present and our future.

It is a work that analyses not only the essence of the human condition, but also how people develop among the growth of personal possibilities. Reading the book, which is both entertaining and profound, is enormously liberating, it manages to infect you with a great enthusiasm and serenity in your daily life. It brings us closer to others in an elegant and profound way.

Reading Zeldin allows us to learn from everything he has studied. It lets us apply the joys of study and curiosity to our lives.

Throughout his life, his curiosity has been applied to the study of specifically French character traits. If Churchill, when asked what the French are like, replied that he could not answer since he did not know them all, perhaps Zeldin has given a voice to a few hundred people to demonstrate the plurality of human life. Since then, he has focused on how work can be made less boring and frustrating, how conversation can be less superficial, and how people can be more honest with their own lives.

d. EVERYDAY REFLECTIONS

After reading his work, we will never be alone again. Zeldin delivers a lifetime of study to us, in which we open ourselves to the great human family. It is not the same as turning on the National Geographic channel. It is to be part of someone who wants to transcend only their own life. It is the humble and empathetic vision of someone giving us the world.

e. OTHER RELEVANT FRAGMENTS

"People who want to be free need to dig over a much wider area, and deeper, to understand their personal emotions and ambitions."

"However, loneliness is not incurable, any more than smallpox is. Its history shows that some people have developed more or less immunity from it by four methods. What these methods have in common is that they have followed the principle on which vaccination works, using loneliness itself, in calculated doses, to avoid being destroyed by it."

"The pioneers were the hermits. They were men and women who felt out of place in the world, who did not like its greed cruelty and compromises or who believed they were misunderstood."

"The retreat often turned the original Hindu idea back to front, making it a preparation for life rather than death."

"The second form of immunisation against loneliness involved not moving out of society, nor searching for God, but turning inwards, with the aim of reinforcing one's powers of resistance, through introspection, the understanding of oneself, by emphasising one's uniqueness, even though at first that might increase the loneliness."

"The third way of tolerating loneliness was by an injection of the absurd. British eccentrics combined loneliness with humour and extracted courage from the mixture. Eccentrics have sadly tended to be left out of history books, which have a misplaced idea of what it means to be serious."

"The final form of immunisation has been achieved by thinking that the world is not just a vast, frightening wilderness, that some kind of order is discernible in it, and that the individual, however significant contains echoes of that coherence."

"It is now clear, therefore, that everyone needs small doses of foreign bodies that in order to survive side by side with others, it is necessary to absorb a minute part of them. It is impossible to cut oneself off, or destroy one's enemies forever. Curiosity about others can no longer be thought of as a luxury or a distraction: it is indispensable to one's very existence."

f. SUGGESTED READING

An Intimate History of Humanity, New York, HarperCollins, 1995.

Conversation. How Talk Can Change Our Lives, London, The Harvill Press, 1998.

The Hidden Pleasures of Life, London, Quercus, 2016.

The return of humanism
Stefan Zweig

a. WHO IS STEFAN ZWEIG?

Stefan Zweig (Vienna, 1881-Petrópolis, Brazil, 1942) was a writer of novels, short stories and biographies written in German. Zweig was the son of a wealthy Jewish family, although he was not educated in Judaism. He received his doctorate in Philosophy from the University of Vienna and thanks to his financial status he was able to travel all over the world to places such as India and the United States, and to live in Salzburg for twenty years. During his life he visited the Soviet Union, lived in London, settled in Zurich and finally moved to Brazil.

During World War I, and after having served in the Austrian Army for some time as an employee of the War Office (he had been declared unfit for combat), he went into exile in Zurich because of his anti-war convictions, influenced by Romain Rolland. He immediately settled in Switzerland. In 1928 he travelled to the Soviet Union. Zweig went on to cultivate friendships with figures such as Máximo Gorki, Rainer Maria Rilke, Auguste Rodin, Arturo Toscanini, Joseph Roth, Hermann Hesse and Albert Einstein.

After the intensification of the National Socialist influence in Austria, Zweig moved to London for a time. By then he began to have difficulties getting published in Germany, but despite this he was able to write the libretto for *Die schweigsame Frau* ('The Silent Woman'), an opera written by composer Richard Strauss.

Defined as "non-Aryan," he was defended by Strauss, who refused to remove Zweig's name as a librettist from the poster for the Dresden-released *The Silent Woman*. Hitler refused to go to the premiere, as planned, and shortly after, following just three performances, the opera was banned.

A humanist and pacifist, he was against the intervention of Germany in the Second World War. In 1934 he began tours of South America. In 1936 his books were banned in Germany by the Nazi regime and in 1938 he divorced his first wife.

The following year he married Charlotte Elisabeth Altmann and, after the start of the war, Zweig moved to Paris. Shortly after, he travelled to England, where he obtained citizenship and settled.

In 1941 he moved to Petrópolis, in Brazil, where, a year later, desperate over the future of Europe and its culture (after the fall of Singapore), and believing that Nazism would spread over the entire planet, on 22nd February 1942, he and his wife committed suicide.

His masterpiece, *The World of Yesterday*, published posthumously, is an elegy for European culture, which he considered was lost forever.

Context: Europe cannot be understood without the weight of the Austro-Hungarian monarchy, which was – for decades –

the cultural centre of the continent. Zweig is the best example of this, along with authors such as Joseph Roth, Franz Kafka or Arthur Schnitzler. One of the most beautiful books which can be read to understand this time is ***1913: The Year before the Storm***, by Florian Illies.

The first half of the 20th century in Europe cannot be understood without the coming together of two worlds as powerful as Judaism and German culture, whose collision, directly and indirectly, changed the course of history and life – and which meant death for many – of millions and millions of people.

To read Zweig is to read a series of books with the most wonderful reflections ever written on two words fiercely opposed; not only, but very particularly, in his time: humanism and power. And perhaps that is why, instead of commenting here on his masterpiece, ***The World of Yesterday***, or the great book on ***Fouché***, or his wonderful little book ***The Eyes of the Eternal Brother***, we will lean towards a book that, when we read it, will make us feel afraid of absolute power: ***The Right to Heresay: Castellio against Calvino***.

b. FRAGMENTS OF HIS WORK

"Of course, there could have been nothing more logical than that the religious revolutionists, Luther, Zwingli and the other theologians of the Reformation, should have united in brotherly fashion upon a unified creed and a unified practice for the new Church. But when have the logical and the natural swayed the course of history? Instead of a worldwide and united Protestant Church, a number of petty Churches sprang up all over the place."

"Spiritual movements always need a genius to initiate them and another genius to bring them to a close. Luther, the inspirer, set the stone of the Reformation rolling; Calvin, the organiser, stopped the movement before it broke into a thousand fragments. In a sense it may be said, therefore, that the Institutio rounded of the religious revolution, as the Code Napoleón rounded off the French."

"Dictatorship is unthinkable and untenable without force. Whoever wants to maintain power must have the instruments of power in his hands; he who wants to rule must also have the right of inflicting punishment."

"People are prone to accept suggestion, not when it comes from the patient and the righteous, but from monomaniacs who proclaim their own truth as the only possible truth, and their own will as the basic formula of secular war."

"With systematic thoroughness, Calvin set to work upon the realization of his plan to convert Geneva into the first Kingdom of God on Earth. It was to be a community without taint, without corruption, disorder, vice or sin; it was to be the New Jerusalem, a centre from which the salvation of the world would radiate. This one and only idea was to embody Calvin's life; and the whole of his life was to be devoted to the service of this one idea."

c. BRIEF COMMENTARY

Zweig enjoyed considerable fame in his lifetime, and now he is being read once again, and appreciated more than ever. He represents humanist hope, a kind of refuge for active dignity.

Castellio against Calvino is a work that analyses the controversy between a good man and a reformist who wielded absolute power, a dogmatic fundamentalist. The fierce, unmasked man of power.

Reading the book both impresses and causes distress, because you can see how power crushes dissent. It is a work that expresses the enormous force (and fury, in this case) with which Protestantism was expressed; the great counter-power against Catholicism.

In any case, Protestantism versus Catholicism is not all we are reading about here. We are reading about how Calvin applied what we all know, expressed here in the words of Zweig, "With time, authority cannot be exercised without applying violence."

And in this great work we will learn from violence, in a disturbing way.

Here is an opportunity to delve a little deeper into this book – and in an extraordinary way – into the human soul.

d. EVERYDAY REFLECTIONS

To read Zweig is to understand applied geography and history. It is to bring to life the time and the place in which we live. It is to understand that the world is not only ours. It is to pause and feel like our other lives. It is to incorporate humanistic reflection within a historical context. It is to feel vertigo with everything that disappears. It is to value what we are, what we had, what we could be. And it is, therefore, to appreciate our lives.

Reading Zweig in a state of tranquillity, will, at the same time, put you in a state of alert. It humanises your perspective. It makes you read the news and the world knowing all that can be lost when the tectonic plates of geography and history begin to shift.

e. OTHER RELEVANT FRAGMENTS

"Tolerance versus intolerance, freedom versus tutelage, humaneness versus fanaticism, individuality versus mechanical uniformity, conscience versus violence. [...] these names signify and inward and personal decision as to which counts more for us: mankind or politics, the ethos or the logos, personality or community."

f. SUGGESTED READING

The World of Yesterday: Memoirs of a European, London, Pushkin Press, 2011.

Shooting Stars: 10 Historical Miniatures, London, Pushkin Press, 2015.

Joseph Fouché: Portrait of a Politician, Lexington, Plunkett Lake Press, 2012.

The Right to Heresay: Castellio against Calvino, Lexington, Plunkett Lake Press, 2015.

The Eyes of the Eternal Brother, Austin, Press Intermezzo, 2003.

The embodiment of wisdom and compassion

The Buddha, by Agustín Pániker*

a. WHO IS THE BUDDHA?

Siddhartha Gautama, who later became known as "The Awakened One" (the Buddha) or the "Sage of the Shakyas" (Sakyamuni), must have lived between 520 and 440 BC, although there is little certainty about his biographical traits.

Legend has it that he was the crown prince of the small kingdom of Shakya, north of India and south of Nepal. After spending his childhood and adolescence at the palace, at the age of twenty-nine he decided to give up a life guided by ignorance, the fulfilment of traditions and a future as a monarch, and dedicate himself to the inner search, focusing on how to end the inherent suffering of the human condition. After six years of searching with the yogis and ascetics of ancient India, it is said that – in his intense meditations – he awoke to reality as it is: transitory, contingent, lacking in substance and void of its own nature. He found the "middle way" (between the hedonistic way of the palace and the mortifications of ascetic practices) that leads to the peace of nirvana.

* The publisher of Editorial Kairós.

Out of compassion, he decided to proclaim his vision and the path that leads to freedom near the city of Benares. After his first sermon and the conversion of five disciples, the Buddhist community was formed. For the next forty-five years, the Buddha and his followers preached the "middle way" all over the Ganges valley. His message appealed to the nobility, the new urban merchant collectives, and even Brahmins, who were all tired of the ritualism of Hindu religiosity. At the age of eighty, the Buddha passed away peacefully, surrounded by his disciples and leaving no successor.

From then on, the cult of the Buddha would begin (in the form of the stupas or reliquary milestones that represent him; and later the images) and the transmission of his teaching (through the sutras or orations that contain his word, first orally and then written).

Context: The Buddha is a paradigmatic figure of what has come to be called the "Axial Age", when in different places of the Old World – between 800 and 200 BC. – groups of people (renouncers, sophists, philosophers and even divine avatars) abandoned their social position and the traditions they inherited, to dedicate themselves to a goal beyond human capacity: nirvana, liberation, paradise, God, salvation, atman, Tao, being, and so on. This new spiritual orientation marked a decisive opening of horizons for humanity, when more ethnic or local forms of religious behaviour and thought were abandoned.

The quotes that follow are all from the oldest orations or sutras, originally transmitted in the Pali language (which bears a strong resemblance to Sanskrit) and which probably echo the "word of the Buddha".

b. FRAGMENTS OF HIS WORK

"The disciple Malunkyaputta sees that the master leaves some of the cardinal philosophical questions unanswered (whether the world is eternal or not, whether one exists after death or not, etc.). The Buddha then tells him the following parable:

A man is wounded by a poisoned arrow. His friends rush to find a doctor. When he is about to remove the poisoned arrow from the wounded man, he shouts:

'Halt, I won't let the arrow be taken out of me until I know who it was that shot me: was it a warrior caste man, a Brahmin, a merchant or a commoner; what family and lineage he belonged to; if he was tall, short or of medium height; if he was black, white or yellow skinned…, I will not remove the arrow until I know if the weapon was a bow or a crossbow; if the rope was made of cane, hemp, grass or bark…'

'What would happen, Malunkyaputta?'

'The man would die before all these questions could be answered. In the same way, the disciple who wanted answers to all questions about the afterlife would die before knowing the truth about suffering, the cessation of suffering and the way to end suffering.'"

"'Good Gautama, what is the foundation of the mind?'

'The foundation of the mind is lucid consciousness.'

'And what is the foundation of lucid consciousness?'

'The foundation of lucid consciousness is liberation.'

'And what is the foundation of liberation?'

'The foundation of liberation is nirvana.'

'And what is the foundation of nirvana?'
'This question goes too far, Brahmin. No answer can encompass it.'"

"*Let no one chase the past*
nor live waiting for the future;
because the past is no longer
and the future is yet to be.
What you must look at thoroughly
it is what now arises at every moment."

"*On one occasion the master came across a passerby. Impressed by his peaceful countenance, the traveller inquired:*
'Are you a god?
'No, I am not a god.'
'So, are you a wizard?'
'No, I'm not a wizard.'
'Are you a man?
'No, I am not a man.'
'Then what are you?
'I am awake.'"

"*Lying back and about to enter final nirvana, the Buddha utters his last words: "May each of you be your own island, each your own refuge, without trying to take refuge in any other. May each one of you have teaching as an island, may teaching be a refuge to you."*

c. BRIEF COMMENTARY

The starting point of Buddhist reflection is not cosmological, we are not told about the gods or the creation of the world, since the Buddha was somewhat allergic to metaphysical conjectures (and, in particular, to the notion of an ultimate cause or "God"). So the starting point revolves around an existential problem of the human condition: suffering (encompassing dissatisfaction, alienation, finiteness, stress, contingency, and so on).

And he reveals its cause: ignorance, which impels us to act selfishly and attached, slaves to unhealthy behaviours (which the Buddha encapsulates in the three poisons: greed, hatred and ignorance), apparently as notorious in his time as in ours. To tackle the "disease" he designs a yoga, or spiritual practice (his "middle way", made up of eight members), based on ethical behaviour (focused on non-violence and self-control), on a sapiential understanding (intellectual and experiential) of reality and in some yogic-meditative techniques that facilitate the process.

d. EVERYDAY REFLECTIONS

Nothing the Buddha preaches is theoretical. Its purpose is practical, everyday. The point is to "wake up" from the dream of ignorance and to see things just as they are, that is, without the illusion of an "I" experiencing "things." Nirvana would then be the experience of this world without being dominated by desires, obsessions and attachments. In psychological terms, it would correspond to full adulthood, the self and egoism having been overcome, when one is truly free to act without impulsiveness. A life, in short, of full discernment. In ethical terms, it is the destruction of hatred, evil, greed and nescience. In mystical terms, perhaps it would be the very nature of reality (awakened and conscious), the realisation of oneself, since there is no "enlightened" one. The awakening would not be, then, a breakdown of relationships, but the discovery of a more genuine relationship. That is what the Buddha called "liberation." That is where true freedom lies.

e. OTHER RELEVANT FRAGMENTS

> *"When a practitioner walks, he is aware, 'I am walking.' When he is standing, he is aware, 'I am standing.' When he is sitting, he is aware, 'I am sitting.' When he is lying down, he is aware, 'I am lying down.' The practitioner acts in full awareness in whatever he does."*

> *"Everything that is subject to an origin is necessarily subject to an end."*

> *"Everything that is constituted is impermanent, everything that is constituted involves suffering, everything is without entity."*

> *"To think: 'I am' is an illusion. To think: 'I am this' is an illusion. To think: 'I will be' is an illusion. To think: 'I will not be' is an illusion. Illusions are a disease, a thorn. But he who has left all illusions behind is said to be a 'quiet sage'."*

> *"This life of purity is not practised to acquire fame, honours or profit, nor to achieve a morality, a concentration or perfect knowledge and vision. The definitive liberation of the mind,*

this and only this, is the purpose of the life of purity; its essence,
its consummation."

f. SUGGESTED READING

Essence of the Dhammapada, Tomales, Nilgiri Press, 2013.

El Dhammapada: la senda de la perfección, ('The Dhammapada: The Path of Perfection'), unavailable in English. Barcelona, Plataforma Editorial, 2014.

Majjhima Nikaya: los sermones medios del Buda, ('Majjhima Nikaya: The Central Sermons of the Buddha'), unavailable in English.

The Word of Buddha, Kandy, Buddhist Publication Society, 2016.

We have reached the end of this great little journey on the shoulders of giants, in which we have been able to see further and look even deeper.

We have used books and reading as telescopes and microscopes of our lives.

We have enjoyed the act of reading as a way of thinking. As António Lobo Antunes said, "To think is to listen carefully." In a way, thinking is also to read carefully.

Thank you for joining me on this journey to uncover our souls.

If you can, give yourself a gift: return to your usual bookshop and find a new dose of happiness.

Acknowledgements

To my friend and author Xavier Melgarejo (1963-2017), for teaching me the meaning of "unconditional love"; what he wrote when he came out of his coma. I also greatly appreciate his family's friendship.

To my family, for testing my capacity for unconditional love.

To my team at Plataforma, because there could be more or less of us, but no one better than us.

To my friends, because all the treasures of art and of the spirit would be colourless without your company.

To Xavier Coll, for his generosity and our shared love of reading.

And to Sergio Vila-Sanjuán, Victor Küppers, Santiago Álvarez de Mon and Lluís Bassat, as admired authors and friends. To Daniel Carreño, whom I had the pleasure of meeting at a wonderful conference, thanks to which a magnificent friendship emerged. His words are very generous, and his company is cause for hope for me.

To Luis Alberto de Cuenca, one of the people who enlighten my existence; how lucky I am to be your friend.

To Agustín Pániker, a great editor and friend.

To Sister Paqui Sellés, from the Convento de Carmelitas Descalzas de la Sagrada Familia, in Puçol, for her invaluable help in revising the manuscript.

To the giants on whose shoulders I live: the thirty-three authors cited here – and briefly commented on – would serve to justify a happier life, or, at the very least, a better life, before moving on to a better life.

JORDI NADAL

Your opinion is important.
Your comments are very welcome at:

www.plataformaeditorial.com

Visit your most trusted bookstore.
Having a good bookseller is as recommendable
as having a good doctor.

"I cannot live without books."

THOMAS JEFFERSON

Plataforma Editorial plants a tree
for every title published.

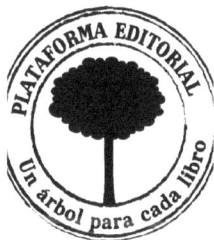

9 781912 914319